THERAPEUTIC
MEDICAL MASSAGE
The Healing Touch

MICHAEL STIERS M.T., B.A.

iUniverse LLC
Bloomington

THERAPEUTIC MEDICAL MASSAGE
THE HEALING TOUCH

iUniverse books may be ordered through booksellers or by contacting:

iUniverse LLC
1663 Liberty Drive
Bloomington, IN 47403
www.iuniverse.com
1-800-Authors (1-800-288-4677)

ISBN: 978-1-4917-2589-4 (sc)
ISBN: 978-1-4917-2590-0 (e)

Library of Congress Control Number: 2014903344

Printed in the United States of America.

iUniverse rev. date: 02/17/2014

CONTENTS

Preface

The subject of Massage Therapy is over whelming as far as the amount of information and subject matter to cover systematically. I have attempted to try to assemble enough information to assist the beginning student and touch on the main aspects of this trade in order to give a good foundation for the novice. Anyone beginning a career in Massage Therapy will eventually evolve to the point where they will develop their own area of expertise, techniques and skill in the many areas of specialization available. This book is a springboard to help in the beginning times when there are so many roads to choose. It is intended to answer basic questions and assist in areas where experience has not been developed with confidence and practice.

There is a basic need for human touch. Compassion for the suffering and understanding is the main tool for a successful practice in this trade. Since I have entered this vocation in 1983 I have learned that there is a reason they call it a practice. Every day you practice and learn something new and are astonished by this wonderful creation we call the human body. The rewards are great when you replace the look of anguish and pain with a smile by just pushing a button on the body.

The secrets of healing and their answers are already inside our bodies. They were made to last an eternity. Our bodies are trying to restore and heal themselves, listen to it, restore the balance, because all they need is a little help. Decades will pass and we will learn and uncover the secrets of repair to heal the human body. I feel there will always be a place for massage therapy. Massage is not invasive, and promotes the basic repair and recovery technique that the body needs. It is my hope that you the student, will continue to add to this knowledge, hone your skills as a healer, and be a credit to the craft.

DEDICATION

This book is dedicated to two wonderful women in my life, my daughter Mickie, and my late wife Debby. My daughter's love for literature and her endless trail of books led her to the profession of librarian and for all of those hours sitting at the L&K eating our breakfast after church going through countless flash cards to help prepare me for the State Medical Boards.

My wife Debby, who has recently gone home to be with the Lord, was a constant source of encouragement, support, and understanding for me. Her wit and smile would melt away the pain she suffered and from filled me with the determination to accomplish any task I planned. Debby always believed in me.

The love and devotion of these two ladies have made me a better man.

CHAPTER 1

What is Therapeutic Massage?

When you manipulate the muscle, tendons, ligaments and fascia of the body in order to restore these soft tissues to what we would consider normal condition, you are performing therapeutic massage. If your goal is to restore the flow of blood, remove waste product and increase the range of movement in the body you are using massage therapeutically. The following is the result of medical massage.

- Charlie Horses and cramps are reduced or removed
- Muscle becomes more pliable, with increased range of motion
- Enhance the fluid movement of the body
- Relaxing the mind and remove stress that tightens soft tissue
- Increase efficiency of breathing
- Aid in the lymphatic movement with increased circulation of blood
- Remove mental trauma that lends itself to headaches, traumatized ligaments and general reduction of pain and inflammation from injury
- Helps to remove scar tissues following surgery or injury
- Improvement in the skin nourishment
- Improvement in posture through changing tension patterns that affect posture
- Massage helps the skin by nourishing it and keeping it plyable
- Massage give you an all over feeling of well being
- Lowers the level of nervousness
- It tunes you in to your body awareness
- Clears your mind and makes tunes you into your body and what is happening
- Relax the stiffness in tight muscle

The clinical benefits of massage therapy has been documented for a long time to help pulmonary functions, chronic inflammatory bowel disease, remove stress, improve depression, and the list goes on and on. In some of the more progressive hospital, infant massage is administered to help the cesarean baby to finish the birthing process. Without the benefit of the contractions experienced in the birthing canal, neural pathways sometimes are not established in the development of the brain. The benefits of massage extend to patients suffering from TMJ, sports injury, depression, digestion problems, arthritis, allergies, anxiety, myofascial pain, headaches, and even insomnia.

Massage Therapy, a brief history

The Chinese were doing massage almost 4000 years ago. During the time of Hippocrates, the "The Father of Medicine", 80% of his practice was the art of rubbing.

The very beginning of our massage we use today was started by Henrik Ling by the turn of the 18th century. This Swedish pioneer developed a system of hard and soft techniques. He later went on to establish The Royal Central Gymnastic Institute in Sweden that taught his methods.

The United States had massage therapy introduced to it in the mid 19th by the Taylor brothers that were New York doctors and educated in Sweden. After the Civil War, two doctors from Sweden opened massage therapy clinics in Boston, (The Posse Institute by Dr. Posse), and another in Washington D.C., the Swedish Health Institute, by Dr. Nissen.

Massage has progressed to many styles or techniques, depending on the expected outcome or goal. The movement and or changing the state of the soft tissues consists of techniques that include ischemic stationary or slow sliding pressure, holding, and/or enabling or restoring motion of or to the body. Massage therapy is performed primarily with the hands, sometimes the forearms or elbows and electric vibrators. These techniques affect the muscles, skeleton, lymphatic, blood flow, nerves, and other systems of the body. The basic goal of massage therapy is assisting the ability of the body to repair itself. It is just a matter of pushing the right buttons and the body can mend as it was intended.

Touch is the fundamental medium of massage therapy. While massage can be described in terms of the type of techniques performed, touch is not used solely in a mechanical way in the therapy. One could look at a drawings, or photos of a massage procedures how to place your hands and what direction the stroke should go or how hard to push, and so on. There is more to giving a massage than memorizing movements and strokes. You must develop palpation skills to the point of feeling the patients pain up to seven layers deep and knowing when the muscle releases. To get results you must consider massage an art.

Massage is done by applying touch with varying levels of pressure and sliding slowly. The massage therapist must adjust the touch and duration of timed pressure with delicate attention in order to determine the optimal amount of pressure, as it varies for each patient depending upon the integrity of the soft tissues for each person. For example, using too much pressure may cause the muscle to tighten up, or too little may not have enough effect. Touch used with an educated palpation skill enables the therapist to feel the tissues that need to be released and where the pain is. After some experience, the therapist can identify the injured soft tissues as much as 7 layers deep. There is a notable difference in the texture of the muscle, the density is usually greater and a noted change in the temperature from the adjacent tissues. The traumatized soft tissues will be hotter for new injuries and colder for an older injury because of the lack of blood flow. This tool provides useful information as far as where the pain is and when the muscle releases. Healing does not take place without intent. It doesn't work by just going through the numbers, the tissues will tolerate just so much and you need to learn to work with the tissue so it won't respond to the treatment as another injury.

In practice many massage therapists use more than one technique. Friction is used on the superficial layers of muscle and in the general direction of the flow of blood toward the heart. Combine it with active and passive movements of the joints to clean out the debris, increase range of motion, and generally tailor the massage session to meet the needs of the patient. Swedish massage is most commonly used.

When you release a muscle there is a noticeable movement that accompanies it and is felt by both the patient and the therapist. It is similar to the sensation of a high density area becoming softer and smaller as if the air is being released out of a balloon. This area becomes smaller and it becomes difficult to keep your thumb on as it tends to roll away as the surface area being treated becomes smaller there is less area to push on. It has been said that healthy tissue can withstand a pressure of 40 lbs. per square inch. Even the surface of the eye when pressed on should not be uncomfortable with that much pressure. In time you will learn to adjust your pressure to adjust to the tissues that you will be working with. Don't try to force it, work with the tissue and the result will be longer lasting. Each patient you work on will differ somewhat as the athlete will be toned and muscle will be harder. When palpated, your will find it difficult to distinguish traumatized muscle or edema when it is well conditioned and toned.

After you develop this ability to find the sore spots and treat them, you may ask what is actually happening and why it does work. This technique is called "Ischemic Compression", (more in depth information will follow later on). In everyday language it means "hurtful pushing". If you use your thumb, elbow or a tool to release a muscle you apply a steady pressure to the belly of the muscle. The belly of the muscle is the middle and widest section as it tapers away to form the tendons on each end. The belly of the muscle is where the nerve from the brain is connected and receives the message to contract. When this area is pressed, the blood is forced out of the capillaries surrounding the nerve endings that are telling the muscle to stay tight. Without the blood, there is no oxygen, and without oxygen the nerve synapse cannot function in order to tell the muscle to be tight. Since there is no impulse from the brain to tell the muscle to contract it relaxes.

Will it last? Why does it take more than one session to repair these injuries and sometimes only one visit for other patients? Every patient presents a new challenge.

Some people have a good response to this treatment. The age, condition and health of your patient, the severity of the injury, not following the suggestions of the therapist for post treatment recovery, genetic engineering, diet habits, are all reasons for slow recovery.

Your patient and you should be considered a team when working together for a solution to their health. There are times when more than one treatment is needed to fix an injury. After the first session maybe half the pain is gone yet there is still range of motion problems and some pain to deal with. You should not work on an injury beyond the "good hurt" stage and cause undo pain even when the patient requests it just to get it over with. You will accomplish more if you work with the body and not beyond what it will tolerate. Even though the patient can stand the pain, the traumatized tissues involved will respond to the therapy as a new injury. It is better to wait and see how long the improvement from the treatment will last. Timing is the critical element here. When the patient feels the injury getting hurtful and tightening up again that is the time to schedule and redo the therapy again. Typically the result will last twice as long as it did the first time. If it returns again the timing is the same, when it hurts again schedule a new treatment. If multiple sessions are required, you will note that you can become a little more aggressive each time as the progress is noted and the repaired; the injury will eventually stay fixed. The longer the patient has been dealing with the injury, the longer it will take to restore it to normalized condition. If your patient gets relief from a session on your table and it starts to hurt again the mileage from each later treatment becomes longer until it just stays

Why doesn't it get better on its own and why does it take multiple sessions sometimes? If you could see a muscle close up it would look like a bundle of spaghetti. When the brain calls upon a muscle to perform a work load, not every fiber in the muscle moves, but rather just enough to perform the task move and the rest are stationary. We have over 700 sets of muscles in our body and they all have certain tightness or tone that they maintain by the sympathetic nervous system to maintain our posture and other duties.

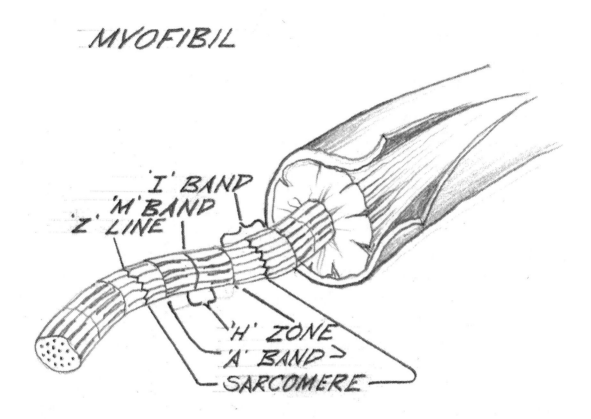

MYOFIBIL

'I' BAND
'M' BAND
'Z' LINE

'H' ZONE
'A' BAND >
SARCOMERE

Some doctors refer to this situation as the muscle memory. This stored spring loaded kinetic energy is accomplished by little bands that go around the fibers called sarcomeres. These sarcomeres have little H bands at intervals. When these H bands line up they attach like Velcro into a holding pattern and when you mechanically dislodge them the muscle fiber slides back to the previous H band that held before. The brain realizes that the muscle is looser and thinks that the tension is to weak. It wants to restore the muscle to its established tone during the injury interval period because it thinks that is the normal tone. With multiple treatments the brain is trained to keep it at this lesser tightness and eventually considers it the correct or normal tightness. We refer to this process neuromuscular re-education.

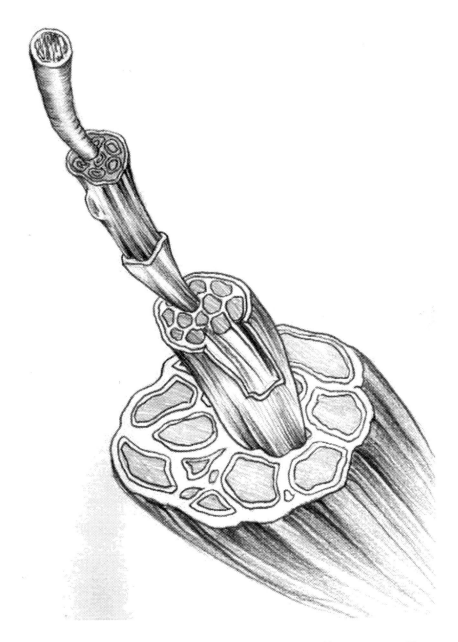

This muscle fiber is like a handful of spaghetti noodles. Many fibers make up the entire muscle wrapped in a fascia membrane. This membrane allows the individual fiber to slide adjacent to the neighboring fiber without getting caught. Not every fiber moves back and forth but just enough to accomplish the work load the brain calls for.

CHAPTER 2

The Massage Table:

One of the most important purchases you will make is your table. You should consider whether your table should be portable or a permanent location in your treatment room. Portable tables are lighter and usually come with a carry case to travel on site. He legs are foldable; you can determine the width and usually the thickness of the padding. I find that too much padding can affect your pressure adversely and suggest it not be too plush. I suggest that you include a headrest that can be attached with a arm sling under it to support the arms. Some tables have a opening to accommodate pregnant women and The

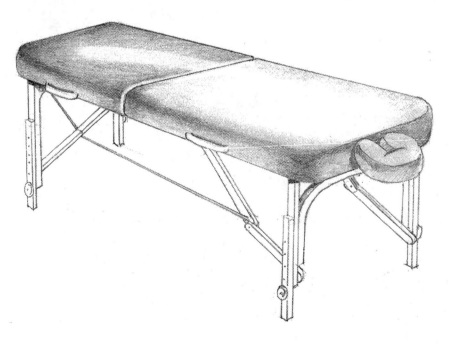

stationary table is heavier and has adjustment for leg height with storage under it for towels and other accessories. Your table height should be adjusted to such a height to allow for the average girth or thickness of your patient and the length of your arms so that when you lean forward to apply pressure you are not bent forward too much to maintain good body mechanics and not tire your back. Like most purchases you should not skimp or a cheap quality as this item will last you many years. Tables can be re-upholstered after years of use when the covering starts to crack and separate.

Oils:

Massage therapy oils are everywhere and easy to find on the market today. You will eventually decide upon your favorite after trying the many varieties. Some have additives included in them to accomplish exfoliation to remove the dead skin. Your oil is used sparingly to facilitate a silky glide without being too slick to move the tissues in the way you need to. A good home made recipe is 5 parts olive oil, 3 parts baby oil, 1 part witch hazel (for disinfectant for those patients who have a lot of body hair) and enough lavender oil to scent it. The lavender achieves a relaxed state mind and it isn't too much of a perfumed aroma for the men.

CHAPTER 3

An Overview of Massage Styles

Swedish massage

Swedish massage uses a system of long gliding strokes, kneading, and friction techniques on the superficial layers of muscles, generally in the direction of the heart, and combines it with active and passive movements of the joints. It is used to promote general relaxation, improve circulation and range of motion, and relieve muscle tension. Swedish massage is the most commonly used and best known type of massage. During Swedish massage the therapist uses massage oils to facilitate smooth gliding strokes called effleurage. Other classic Swedish massage moves include kneading, friction, stretching, wringing, percussion, and sometimes tapping. I have used this method for my general hour massage and when needed switch to deep tissue work on trouble spots as I find them.

A firm but gentle pressure is used to promote relaxation, ease muscle holding patterns, with many other benefits. The biggest benefit is the movement of blood and improvement of circulation, muscle tone, balance of the muscular-skeletal systems, lymph movement, removes toxins and increase oxygen to the cells. An hour of massage does the same thing that it takes your body to do in 8 hours of sleep per night. Therapeutic Massage is used in place of Swedish massage in many situations because it is used to restore medical abnormalities, and regarded by many states and doctors as a reliable, serious branch of alternative medicine. Therapeutic Massage can be preformed on a massage chair as well as a table for shorter sessions or on site.

Aroma Therapy

A complimentary medium for healing that you can use with your massage therapy is aroma therapy. It is a alternative medicine that applied topically to the skin to introduce essential natural healing plant oils that contain chemicals to promote healing and ease. These oils give off a strong and pleasant aroma. Aromatherapy offers diverse physical and mental benefits, depending on the essential oil or oil combination and your method of application used. The medicinal properties of essential oils used in aromatherapy include: analgesic, antimicrobial, antiseptic, anti-bacterial, anti-microbial, anti-inflammatory, astringent, sedative, antispasmoic, expectorant, diuretic, and sedative. These essential oils can be used to treat a wide rage of problems, including, but not limited to gastrointestinal discomfort, skin conditions, menstrual pain and irregularities, stress-related problems, mood disorders, circulatory problems, respiratory infections, and wounds. Aromatic plants have been employed for their healing, preservative and wonderful qualities throughout recorded history all over the world. As early as 1500 B.C. the ancient Egyptians used waters, oils, incense, resins and ointments scented with botanicals for their ceremonies and mummifying. Many countries used the spices and oils for monitory exchange.

As far back as 2700 B.C. the Chinese were aware of the healing properties of essential medicine of India called Ayurveda treated with healing oils. The Greeks and the Romans used fragrances in their baths and for their healing qualities. A French chemist Gattefosse published *his* book on aromatherapy, and introduced in Europe aromatherapy as a medical discipline. Gattefosse, who was employed by a French perfume maker, discovered the healing properties of lavender oil quite by accident when he suffered a severe burn while working and used the closest available liquid, lavender oil, to soak it in.

The herbs and their oils are selected for their combined or singular effect for strong psychological and healing properties. The oils are absorbed through the skin into the blood stream, or olfactory glands. The blood stream picks it up and delivers throughout the body. The strength of an oil, or the how fast it evaporates in open air is thought to be linked to the specific psychological effect of that oil. As a rule of thumb, oils that evaporate quickly are considered to be good for emotionally uplifting, while slowly evaporating ones are thought to be calming. http://medical-dictionary.thefreedictionary

Deep tissue massage

This procedure is best for chronic problems in soft tissue. Much more pressure is used on the muscles that are deep with a sustained pressure. Friction going against the muscle fiber's grain and the release of trigger points as well. This is why it is called deep tissue and unlike Swedish it's deep and more aggressive. Focus is on one isolated area at a time. This is effective for chronic muscular tension. Deep Tissue work helps reduce chronic tension from the body muscles through use of slow strokes and deep finger pressure. The most important use of the deep tissue massage is for the people involved in physically demanding professions like athletics or those suffering from physical injuries. It has been found to be helpful particularity in case of chronically tense areas like stiff necks, sore shoulder and tightness in the low back. It is the best massage for people with muscular pain.

Deep Tissue Massage is most effective for long standing pain, range of motion or mobility problems, repetitive injuries, strains, osteoarthritis pain, fibromyalgia pain, and postural problems. As a matter of fact, the New England Journal of Medicine recommends that it be used for Fibromyalgia pain treatment. Some precautions should be noted as follows:

- Neither the therapist or the patient must not have any infectious skin disease or rashes
- If you have had Chemotherapy or surgery deep tissue work is a bad idea
- Ask your patient if they are prone to blood clots
- Check with the patient's doctor if she is pregnant
- If your patient has burses, open wounds, a hernia or broken bone do not do deep tissue work.

Sports massage

Sports massage techniques that are similar to Swedish and deep tissue, but are specifically adapted to enhance athletic performance, or to repair injuries to improve the training performance and expedite the repair of damaged tissues from the sport.

Acupressure

This is a massage-like therapy similar to acupuncture. However, pressure is applied to the specific points within the acupuncture meridians with the finger or thumb, and not with acupuncture needles. Like neuromuscular massage, acupressure is designed to help relieve painful symptoms and also works to bring balance to the body and mind.

The system applies a finger or thumb pressure to specific points located on the acupuncture meridians (channels of energy flow identified in Asian concepts of anatomy) in order to release blocked energy along these meridians that cause physical discomforts, establish "chi" replenish the flow of negative and positive energy or to re-balance the energy flow.

Shiatsu:

Shiatsu is a Japanese term from the rood words *shi* (fingers) and *atsu* (pressure). Shiatsu is an applied system of massage which is much like acupuncture, try's to unblock and establish the flow of energy, known as *Qi* (*chi* in Chinese, *ki* in Japanese), throughout the body. Shiatsu uses several massage techniques, such as pressing, sweeping, rotating and patting. Moe than techniques, however, shiatsu has been described as a dance, a communication between practitioner and client, grounded in traditional Chinese medicine, ideas and traditions. Included was the study of energy pathways called meridians and the relation of the five elements, earth, water, fire, wood, and metal.

Cranial-Sacral Therapy:

Cranial-Sacral Therapy, or CST, is performed to aid and assist in the circulation of the cerebral fluid that engulfs the nervous system. Predominately brain, brain stem and cranial bones. This procedure requires a very sensitive intuitive touch that takes time to develop. The purpose is to restore rhythmic natural movement that exists between the bones of the skull. Cranial Sacral Therapy is a technique based on Cranial Osteopathy. Like Cranial Osteopathy, Cranial Sacral Therapy seeks to restore the natural rhythmic movement found between the bones of the skull. It does the same for the movements of the sacrum. The purpose of this is to aid the circulation of the cerebral fluid throughout the central nervous system.

Different types of massages.

There are diverse numbers of massage techniques that can be combined or used separately depending on the needs of the individual. For those with Cohn's disease for example, some massage therapies that may be used include but are not limited to:

Swedish massage—This is the most common massage used in North America and is characterized by long smooth motions, kneading or applying friction to the surface of the muscles. This type of massage encourages overall relaxation, improves circulation, and relieves tension within the muscles.

Deep tissue massage—This massage involves the use of deep slow stroking motions, friction, or direct pressure to the muscles. Intense pressure is applied for this massage to penetrate deeper into the muscles. It helps relieve chronic muscle tension.

Neuromuscular massage—This massage focuses on the deep penetration of individual muscles. Its purpose is to increase blood flow and release knots of tension that exist in muscles connected to other areas of the body where pain is present. The release of this muscle tension often reduces painful symptoms.

CHAPTER 4

Massage is healing

Massage Therapy is rapidly becoming a leading form of healing in today's society. It has been one of the oldest forms of healing and used all over the world. There is a need for human touch. Most babies stop their crying when picked up and stroked. The first instinct when you hurt yourself is to rub it and massage it. This soothing instinctive touch is usually helpful and we all have this built in action of taking away the "ouch" with a gentle pressure and flexing the sore spot immediately after an injury. Why does this make us feel better?

When we hurt ourselves, the first instinct is to start rubbing the pain. Our bodies automatically know what it wants and without thinking you perform this primal instinct. It brings into the area new blood which helps to remove the histamine and re know place it with anti-histamine to reduce edema or swelling. In addition, the new blood carries away debris and waste buildup to deliver repair materials to the injury. In addition to these actions the blood brings into the area endorphins that are the body pain killer to help deal with the pain. No healing can take place in the body without the blood. There is no condition that the body deals with a far as disease, injury, or any malfunction that can heal without the blood. The blood is the basis of all healing in the body and massage therapy enhances the circulation to set up an environment to restore normal conditions better than any procedure or modality.

There is a lot of joint movement in massage therapy which helps to maintain range of motion, and to pump out the joints that load up with waste product. Since bone tissue has less blood flow the waste accumulates and the joint movement helps to pump and clean the joint so the blood from the massage will carry it away.

The lymphatic drainage is aided by having a massage. An hour's massage does the same thing as 8 hours of sleep can do for the body. The lymphatic system completes a cycle every 12 hours and this process is helped by massage. Detoxifying the body with massage removes debris, toxins, waste material, meds, and much more unwanted materials.

The skin benefits greatly from frequent massage. The aging process is slowed down with the delivery of blood to nourish the skin. The skin of the face is the only place on the body where the muscle is attached to it. The facial expressions are possible because of this. Regular facials can actually tone up the muscle and keep a youthful firm look of the skin and slow down the wrinkle development. Facial massage can manage moisture problems, eliminate oily spots, cleanse the pores and lift sagging muscle.

Massage therapy can help immensely with stress. Most people consider stress to be a traumatic situation like a surgery, death of a friend, divorce etc. Stress is anything that upsets the homeostasis of the body by definition. Homeostasis is the peaceful tranquility like a mirror finish lake. When someone throws a pebble in the lake the ripples start spreading until they hit the bank and disappear. Everything in our body works together to keep this homeostasis, a loud noise and our heart beasts faster, the erector pili muscles of each hair stands them up; our muscles flex or perhaps make us jump. Your setting at a stop light and your in a hurry to get to your destination and your tapping your foot waiting for that long awaited green light and when it finally does change you forget about it and deal with the situation at hand. Our Sympathetic Nervous System tightens up a group of muscles from our neck at the sub-occipital, and spreading down the cervical area the Trapezoids, and down between the scapulas. These soft tissues contract as the brain dumps these daily life mini traumas into this area. The more stress the tighter they get. Actually these muscles are doing their job and without this process you would have a nervous breakdown. Some people grind their teeth at night and other keep in their stomach and develop ulcers. We all have our ways to de-stress and massage is one of the best.

Massage is used in Hospice to relax and help subdue the pain and discomfort of the patient. Equestrian massage is used to repair damage to the horses today. Massage is used in some of the more progressive hospitals to help the new born infants that arrived cesarean style finish the birthing process by simulating the contractions of the birth canal.

Relaxation massage is one of the best gifts to someone you love to pamper them and tell them they are special and is also used as a gift for family members and special friends.

Sports massage is used in the Olympics to prepare the athlete for competition and help recover from the competition.

Massage can do many things to eliminate surgery, one can drain a gall bladder, straighten a coccyx, maintain spacing for the Nucleus Pulpous to recede back into a disc, re-locate an organ that has been moved from a accident, TMJ (Temporal Mandibular Joint Dysfunction), headache pain, Torticolis Wry Neck Syndrome, Sciatic pain, back pain, Scoliosis and many more.

Hippocrates is considered to be the father of medicine that we know today and his procedures for healing consisted of 85% massage and manipulation and the rest being herbs and elicitors. Massage has been around for a long time and it looks like its here to stay.

CHAPTER 5

How Muscular Skeletal Pain Spreads

Muscle spasms and cramps can be very painful. Sometimes muscles can cramp up so bad that they leave a bruise. These involuntary contractions in the muscle do not release and need some help. This requires lengthening the muscle manually. These tight muscles usually occur in the legs and feet where a muscle crosses over a joint as in the calf usually the Gastrocnemius or Soleus muscles and even at times all of the soft tissue muscle in a group. When contracted, these muscles feel rock hard and last from only a few seconds to many minutes. They may return after easing up and then return several times.

Some reasons as to why this happens are: exercising in very hot conditions and the perspiration remove electrolytes like salt, potassium, magnesium and calcium. Dehydration and loss of electrolytes result in loss of muscle control and coordination. Poor conditioning and using the muscles in a new way or activity also contributes to cramping. Excess Lactic Acid build up after exercising also contributes to this condition.

Prevention of cramps can be as simple as improving your fitness level, stretching before and after exercise, or simply maintain your mineral balances in your system. One easy way to accomplish this is to take more magnesium. The "Holy Grail" of all of your minerals is Magnesium. All of your minerals in the body key off of Magnesium. For example, your body maintains a ratio of twice as much Calcium to Magnesium. If you take Calcium to raise the level to the desired amount, it will not increase since the Magnesium is low and stores the additional

Calcium in the fat cells. If you increase the Magnesium to the desired level all of the other minerals will maintain their proper levels automatically since they key off the Magnesium. Magnesium is water soluble and will not build up. Your body will remove the excess through the urinary track and not overdose.

A good example of skeletal pain is when a muscle is repeatedly required to do a repetitive movement, excess resistance in moving a work load, as in weight lifting, range of motion limitation, and some injuries require intense pressure on the skeletal system. When a tendon attachment to the bone becomes traumatized, the brain senses this weakness and builds up re-enforcement to strengthen the area. This condition is called a bone spur. Tremendous torque is used when one just raises the body up on the balls of the foot. This action causes the calf muscle to lift 3 times your body weight as the calf muscle is considered a 3rd class lever, which is the most inefficient lever. The attachment of the Achilles tendon that is attached to the Calcanial Bone is so tight the Pariosteum, (the skin of the bone) becomes bruised and your heal hurts. The bone spur will return after surgical removal because the reason for its existence is not removed in most cases. If the muscles in the calf are lengthened, the stress on the bone is removed and the spur diminishes.

CHAPTER 6

Referred Pain

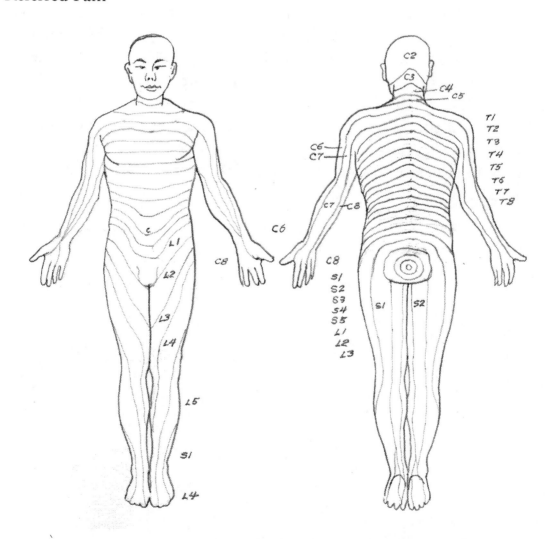

Dermatomes: Derma is the Latin derivative for skin, and tone means area. These skin areas reflect discomfort and pain that do not always originate from the site of the pain. After trying to release the muscles in the area of distress and the results do not change the level of pain after repeated attempts, consider this situation a dermatome area. One example is gall bladder pain that may refer to the back near the scapula. The nerve that leads to the gall bladder is also reflected to the skin in the area near the right scapula.

This referred pain can extend to other areas of the body even though it's origin is nowhere near the culprit. When the Periformis presses onto the Sciatic Nerve the pain can extend all the way down to the great toe of the same leg. great toe where it ends. This nerve is quite large, (the size of your thumb) and is usually traumatized by muscle edema of the Periformis. Nerves originate from the spinal cord and are either sensory or motor nerves. The sensory nerves give sensations to skin (dermatomes) patterns and give clues as to where the problem originates.

The nerves that correspond to the spinal cord as it descends downward in the list below may be helpful to locate the dermatomes responsible for the discomfort.

Location of Pain/Dermatome	Nerve at Spine
Shoulders	C4, C5
Forearms	C6, T1
Thumb and Little Fingers	C6, C7, C8
Thigh Fronts	L2
Side and Mid Calves	S1

Do you remember when your doctor tapped your knee to see if it caused your leg to slightly kick forward? Sometimes he would poke an area with something slightly sharp to see if the nerve responds. If the result is not what he expects then there is an indication of an abnormal nerve response. The lack of response indicates nerve damage, or disruption caused by impingement upon the nerve. If the tendon does not respond, the nerve that activates it could be the reason. The root nerve starting at the cervical spinal cord could be the reason. Tendon reflexes can be checked by the following guide.

Reflex test Area	Spine Nerve Location
Bicepts	C5, C6
Forearm	C6, C7
Triceps and Elbow	C7
Stomach	T8, T9, T10, T11, T12,
Thigh, Knee	L3, L4
Ankle	S1

If you use more pressure and hold it for a little longer on the trigger point you are using deep tissue technique. After developing your palpation skills, you will be able to tell the trigger points easier. After finding these areas you move very slowly along the fibers and connective tissues as you feel the fibers collapse under your pressure. Scar tissue and adhesions develop after injuries or surgery and this method is helpful to break them up.

This style of massage uses a technique called "Ischemic Compression". From the Latin root meaning painful pushing. When pressure is applied to the area the blood is pushed out and therefore the oxygen is also removed. The function of the nerve synapse cannot be completed without oxygen. The signal sending "ouch" to the brain cannot be completed and the cycle of pain diminishes.

This therapy is focused on the deep layers of muscle, tendons, ligaments, and surfaces of the bone. The range of motion can be restored by breaking up scar tissues, and restoring blood circulation to the damaged area. The blood has a tendency to travel around the affected painful areas and waste products accumulate perpetuating this condition. Restore the circulation and you cleanse the area, remove debris, Histamine that causes edema, and brings in anti-Histamine to remove swelling, brings in repair material, and your body's natural pain killers encephalon's and endorphins. Stretching and elongation of the extremities enhances the deep work. Pressure should be forceful enough to produce a so-called "good hurt". Some patients will say "Go ahead and get it out of there, I can take it." If you are too aggressive with your force, the tissue will respond to the therapy like a new injury. You catch more flies with honey and you will learn to adopt your force accordingly to the resilience and tone of the patient. Obese patients require less pressure and an athlete can endure more. Someone with good physically conditioned toned muscle is more difficult to the tissues.

Usually after a serious injury the time worked on the sore areas and pressure is less intense and the next massage session can be more intense and aggressive. As the injury improves the tolerance of receiving the massage becomes a little more forgiving and received better. After each session the time interval should be further apart when finally the muscle stays released and in a state of normality. Deep tissue work is more useful on the larger muscle masses like the hips, and thigh area. Since these muscles are large they require more pressure and deeper penetration to accomplish the results. Apply enough pressure to feel like a good hurt for lack of a better description. After the invasion of such traumatized soft tissues you should end with some gentle friction which helps to soothe the pain. Most patients see even more results after the dust settles from the invasion of you working on a sore area.

CHAPTER 7

The Role of the Therapist

When a patient receives a massage or therapy from you they have put their confidence in you. They respect and trust you. They confide in you, and sometimes you are the only person they have to talk to and share their life. Sometimes you are the only person to share their thoughts if they are an elderly person, family is not near or just one who has few friends. This role should not be taken lightly and the relationship of your patient/ therapist should not only be professional but private. You don't share other people's lives and confidence with other people. Respect the privacy and health condition.

People become comfortable with you and your style similar to the relationship they have with their barber or hair stylist and do not like to change. They look forward to spending quiet time and reward themselves to the comfortable setting in your treatment room environment. It helps to remember each person's preferences. Some like a pillow or a headrest some prefer a blanket for warmth, certain styles of music for background, and some prefer not to talk at all.

Professionalism promotes respect and credibility in the craft. You should dress to look like a professional, your hygiene should be above standard, attention to your nails and hands are the utmost concern. Don't be afraid to explain the reason for your particular treatment and what is happening to the patient's body. Educate them as you go along and give them an idea what to expect with plan of healing. You and your patient are a team and should work together towards restoring normality and optimum health. Remember you patients background, names of family members and the type of work they do for conversation and a tool for assessment of the injury if work related. If they have any recreation passions you are aware of, it can help to diagnose the reasons for injury and help to eliminate them again.

The longer you are in practice the skill level increases as well. Make it a habit to increase your knowledge and continue to extend your level of education. Take classes to widen your knowledge, zero in on new techniques, the more tools you have at your disposal the more success you will have in your treatments.

It has been said, "Out of sight, out of mind." Be involved in your community, they are the ones who patronize you and you need to be in the lime light, get out and drum up business. Have your business cards on you at all times. Take the time to answer questions of people who approach you, establish your credibility and show concern as you network and meet prospective clientele. Don't over book your appointments and be punctual. Keep regular hours and establish solidity with your business. Most of all it is important to treat with intent don't just go through the motions and have your mind somewhere else or it won't work at all. This attitude for the therapist is what I consider the most important one of all. One of the best diagnostic tools that you will have is to listen to your patient.

The reason they call it a practice is that you never stop learning. The rewards are worth it when you see a patient return because he forgot his cane or crutch.

CHAPTER 8

Contraindications for massage

o The first few months of pregnancy
the fetus is very vulnerable during the first three months. Massage during the first trimester will raise the risk of miscarriage. It is generally not considered safe to massage pregnant women, particularly in the first trimester. A very light gentle relaxation massage without any deep pressure or perhaps a fascial to reduce stress is acceptable.

o Fever
Massage releases toxins and free radicals for elimination. If your patient is fighting infection of any kind it already has enough to deal with so don't add to the problem if the immune system is fighting an invader.

o Bruises, incisions, cuts or wounds that are open
Use gentle friction around the concerned area to help the blood supply remove wastes and bring in repair material. Direct the blood towards the heart in venous flow. Apply only light touch drainage massage around the site, to assist the blood flow towards the heart and encourage healing where bruising is present. Oil can contaminate on open areas of the skin. If you have any cuts or open skin area on the hands you should seal them from contamination.

o Hematoma
If you are aware of any danger of blood clot massage is most likely to release the clot or dislodge it causing a stroke. This could also result into a heart attack.

o Thrombosis and varicose veins,
when blood flow is impaired or restricted because of the integrity of the venous structure massage will add to the already backed up flow. These capillaries are already challenged and the blood will most likely coagulate. The heart will also be affected. Light simulative massage over the varicose area will gently break up any coagulation and perhaps aid in the repair of the vessels. Do not massage over broken or varicose veins as the blood supply is impaired in this area. Massage will increase blood flow and flood the over-worked capillaries and veins, possibly causing coagulation and affecting blood flow to the heart after gaining permission from the patient's doctor.

o Contagious skin disorders
Massage can add to the already existing problems if you are dealing with psoriasis, fungus, and viral infections bacterial infection. Always seek the advise of the patient's physician.

o Cancer
Massage can actually help spread the cancer through the lymphatic system, and because massage increases lymphatic circulation, it may potentially spread the disease as well. Gentle caring touch is good, but any stroke that is designed to move blood should not be used, massage strokes that stimulate circulation are not. Always a good idea. Always check with the doctor first and if the prognosis is not good, sometimes a stress reduction gentle massage is the better judgment. In any case it is the doctor's call.

o Broken bones / Fractures
Bones that are mending should be avoided. Light friction to bring into the surrounding area may be helpful to speed up repair and help restore ossification. Too much pressure may reverse the healing process if it is dealing with cancer. Stay away from an area of mending bones.

CHAPTER 9

Effleurage

One of the four basic techniques used is Effleurage. It has technique sub strokes. Some are used for specific medical problems and work on special parts of the body and are chosen for maximum effect. Keep your wrists locked to prevent injury to yourself when using these procedures. Your hand slides over the skin surface with just enough pressure so the skin to form a fold slightly.

Flat Effleurage is done with your hand and fingers level, keeping it loose and no tension. It is used to massage large parts of the body like the back, stomach, chest etc.

Clasping Effleurage is slightly different. The hand is flexed with the thumb not flat but slightly cupped. This method takes on the shape of the body part like the thigh and other extremities, sides of the body buttocks and other parts of the body in a curved shape.

Flat or Clasping Effleurage can be used on the surface or deep depending on your need. If you prefer deep work you need to flex your or stiffen it up to support the increased pressure. This sub stroke is helpful for the lymph and blood circulation. Under deep effleurage pressure the movement of liquid is five times more.

Surface Effleurage has a calming affect on the central nervous system. It removes stress and relaxes the tissues. It improves the function of the vessels, helps the skin tone and elasticity, it stimulates the metabolism of the subcutaneous tissues. Effleurage is usually done with two hands in the direction of the lymphatic and blood flow towards the heart. The hands can be doubled on top of each other for a deeper pressure, or successively repeating the stroke and one at a time following the other.

Be conscious of the direction of your strokes. Push the blood towards the heart when ever possible and know that the lymph vessels move towards the torso of the body.

CHAPTER 10

Lymphatics:

Going against the lymphatic flow reduces the goals of the massage. Most of the initial lymph vessels are located in or just below the skin that drain into larger vessels then into collectors which ultimately drain into the thoracic duct that traverses your chest cavity. There is a suction vacuum effect that helps to move the thick sludge called lymph and is affected by contractions of the muscles and makes a complete cycle twice a day. Pressure from your hand should be just deep enough to be more than sliding over the skin but still not feel the muscles below. One to four ounces of pressure is adequate and too much will actually collapse the vessels and dramatically impede the lymphatic flow for hours. Proper massage technique can increase the flow of lymph as much as 20 times. When the skin is lightly stretched, lymph vessels in the skin first open and then are stimulated to contract and move lymph fluid along. After moving gradually toward the node, relax any pressure you've applied with your fingers—but don't remove your fingers from the surface of your skin. Keeping the fingers in contact with the skin allows the lymphatic valves to close and the lymph to be sucked further down the lymphatic channels.

From the chart, you can see the direction that the lymph needs to move. It's important that you follow the proper direction since forcing lymph in the wrong direction can damage the small lymph vessel valves. It's always best to refer to the drawings since the lymph channels don't flow straight toward the thoracic duct. In draining the different quadrants of the breast, for example, you'll need to massage in different directions.

Where you begin your massaging action is also extremely important. In lymphatic massage always begin your massage nearest to the node that you're draining to. Start about four inches (one hand-width) away from the node and begin to push the lymph toward the node. Continue the process to the end of the line—always pushing the lymph fluid in the direction of the node. This clears the lymph in front of the node so more fluid can move to the node. It also creates suction that pulls more fluid down the path.

Lymphatic drainage is not usually taught in medical school. Improving lymph flow through the massage techniques outlined here can lend great improvement on your health. Some heart doctors even believe that improving the flow and of lymph is now a primary reduction of our heart disease epidemic. Poor lymph circulation can be a good reason for any of these problems: high blood pressure; chronic fatigue; depression; heart problems, rheumatoid arthritis, and weakness or tightness in a limb, skin problems.

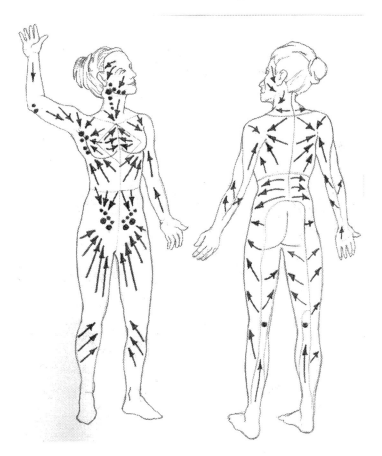

Continuous Effleurage is a seemingly unbroken motion sliding over the skin and relaxes down the nervous system. This is effective over large surfaces where the skin receptors. If the pressure is gradually increased the nerve receptors are not disrupted and become very forgiving readily.

Faltering Effleurage is a simulative method that excites the nervous system, contrary to the affects that effleurage normally does to the nervous system. Activation of the flow of blood by loading the tissues has a warming affect on the muscles. This warmth is caused by the blood brought from the inner core of the body which is a few degrees hotter than the surface blood. This form of effleurage is usually done with athletes and lends itself to the contraction ability of muscle fiber.

Raking Effleurage is like the name implies. Place one hand on the top of the other with the finger tips spread which resembles a leaf rake if you will, and move the soft tissue in the direction desired either sideways or vertical manner. This technique stimulates blood flow, breaks up scar tissue and separates muscle fiber. The movement can be in a circular direction, parallel or vertical.

Stroking Effleurage is done with the knuckles using not too much pressure to excite and wake up muscle fiber. It promotes fiber movement by separating the strands and reestablishing muscle memory by releasing the H bands.

Effleurage is most lost likely the technique that you will use the most. I find that I start the massage session and it is usually the technique that completes it. Effleurage lends itself to one of the main reasons for giving a massage, the blood flow exchange is improved, sweat glands become more efficient, it aids in the absorption for the tissue's nutrients, and improves the integrity of all vessels of the veins, artery, lymph and capillaries. The ability of movement for the muscles is enhanced; it improves elasticity for the skin and muscles, removes the toxins from the epidermis, it removes inflammatory conditions therefore lessening the pain and brings into the system anti-histamine, and calms the nervous system.

The pressure of this method moves blood into the areas desired. The absence of blood also means there is an absence of oxygen. Without oxygen, the nerves can not complete the synapse to tell the muscle to stay tight, and the muscle relaxes because there in no message from the brain to tell it otherwise. The cycle is incomplete and cannot be repeated to keep the pain cycle going. In other words, without oxygen it runs out of gas and gives up the ghost.

CHAPTER 11

Friction

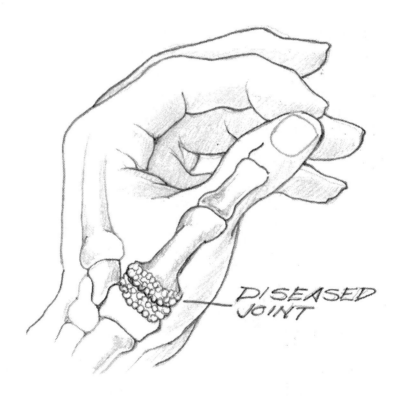

DISEASED JOINT

Friction is done by applying pressure down in a downward direction into the tissues and moves in the desired direction. This motion will create a dent or wrinkle in the skin. There is considerable more force and can be used to separate scar tissue, muscle fiber, movement and stretching of the striated muscle fiber. You may choose to go against or with the grain of the soft tissue worked on. Lock the joints of the fingers that are flexed and do not move during this technique. The wrist is fixed and the force originates from the larger joints such as the elbow and shoulders. Friction movements are usually done the thumbs, although the fingertips, knuckles and the elbow can be used in the sciatica for example). Be sure to use good body ergonomics to preserve the joints in your hand. Over the years of practice without proper precaution you may limit the number of years that you can practice. Some therapist wear out the thumbs and their career is cut short by blowing out your Pollex or also called the Basel joint, (thumb joint). Use your body's weight when leaning and not the muscles of your arm to push with. Lock your thumb joint while leaning over your patient. This allows you to apply pressure constantly and evenly much easier. The healthy body should be able to tolerate 40 lbs. per square inch on any spot of the surface so don't be afraid to apply release pressure

The benefit of this technique is particularly useful for breaking down knots that accumulate in the body from stress caused by the daily life trials and tribulations. Fibromyalgia sufferers will benefit greatly from this method. The fibroblast cells accumulated in the pockets of pain can be broken to restore fiber movement again. Friction helps to break down the waste product from adhesions and a scar tissue, which prevents to scar or adhesion from increased growth. Friction will break up cellulite and fatty deposits and will help with obesity problems. Friction can be effective around scars and adhesions that have formed. Relief of pain temporarily is achieved by the increased cellular activity and accumulation of blood which raises the temperature.

This analgesia effect can be increased in any given area if you use a Russian form of friction by using the edges of your hands (opposite side of the thumb side like a Karate chop position) placed close together and alternating directions with pressure to bring blood from the core of the Mediasteinum where the blood is a couple of degrees higher.

As you work on the muscle with friction, don't force your way into it. You will develop your palpation skills and feel the muscle drop or flatten out if you will as it releases. I remember the days in collage when an instructor said that you will develop palpation skills and be able to feel the target site up to 7 layers of tissue deep and know which direction the fibers go. You will feel hot spots from recent injury and cold spots from older injuries. Follow up with a stroking to help move out any waste product that you released and removes it. Work deeper as you feel the tissue release and become more pliable, then deeper again as you feel the tissue flatten out.

Transverse Friction is applied when you go across the fiber direction of the muscles. Most transverse friction massage techniques are easy to perform, but one needs to respect some technical details. Exact positioning is imperative so that deep friction is given at the site of the lesion; this is where you need to address the scar formation and break it up. The friction needs to be applied in and on the structure beneath the skin. Do not glide over the skin but use a firm deep penetration to the target site with a cross fiber movement. The depth of the friction is sufficient. How deep you go depends upon the location of the structure. Concentrate on making an arm movement instead of a finger pressure movement. Keep the finger joint flexed so it will not bend. The movement consists of two phases, one with pressure and pause after about 10 seconds of pressure then let up for about 5 seconds. For most strains or lesions, approximately 3 times a week should suffice. Friction is more effective without lubricant. The skin is designed to move freely over the muscle while the muscles are able to glide over each other freely without tangling. This is accomplished because each muscle, striated or smooth, along with every nerve, organ, veins, and arteries, capillaries etc. are all individually wrapped with their own bag or covering called fascia. When an injury or surgery occurs the fascia is disrupted and adheres to the adjacent fascia and limits movement of the affected soft tissues. This forms a scar. If the body uses the materials from tissue that is not parietal tissue it is called a keloyd. This scar forms during the healing process. This adheres and keeps the fibers from sliding smoothly. The pain of an injury or surgery is the fascia tearing when movement is attempted. The injured area or areas should not exceed 10 to 15 minutes of friction during the treatment. The surrounding soft tissues should be worked first for sympathetic pain treatment and stretching in the joints to accompany the procedure. Friction with effleurage afterwards will help. After improvement is noted, with only a lingering discomfort the treatment can cease. There will be some tenderness that can be ignored upon palpation. Continue treatments on the quadriceps and the hamstrings even after significant pain reduction in order for full recovery.

Fascia is throughout the body. This is a covering that envelopes all muscles both striated and smooth. This also encapsulates all the vessels and organs. Fascia is a translucent bag that isolates these body parts so things can slide and move independently without getting all mixed up. When a muscle is tight the fascia is also tight. Fascia maintains the shape and transmits movement while supporting the muscle fibers. Myofascial release is the term coined for the bodywork pertaining to this. "Myo" is the Latin prefix meaning muscle and fascial pertains to covering.

CHAPTER 12

What does Myofascial Release do?

Basically it is deep tissue work for the purpose of releasing and separating stuck, restricted fascia. This fascia adheres to the muscle fiber and becomes unplayable and stiff in texture. This situation also occurs in response to physical or emotional trauma. Physical injuries, back and neck pain, along with whiplash, stress related muscular tension and repetitive strain injuries. Prolonged situations as mentioned, promotes non-movement, restricts blood flow and the fascia becomes stiff and dehydrated. MFR is also used in the treatment of immune system dysfunctions such as Fibromyalgia. Massage is the number one recommended approach and treatment for Fibromyalgia by the American Medical Association. Scar tissue resulting from surgery is simply the fascia being cut and adhering to the muscle fibers and adjacent fascia. The movement of the muscle fibers trying to perform their functions and tearing free is the recovery pain experienced from fascia pulling free.

Fascia is strong enough to support over 2000 lbs. per sq. inch. Healthy fascia that is not dehydrated can stretch and move freely without tearing or no restrictions. Fascia is continuous throughout the body and basically separates the inside of the body from the outside world in every orifice of the body. Any restriction of the movement of fascia affects other body parts and can cause pain throughout the body.

Fascia that is not resilient or shortened by surgery or accident injury and hard restricts vessels and nerves. The sharp and deep pain felt can be the result of another injury transmitted from another injury via the domino effect so to speak.

Trigger points are areas of muscle fibers within a muscle, which the brain has decided need to be contracted—switched 'on' and shortened. They occur through accidents, falls, injuries, repetitive strain, overuse of muscles and poor posture. Trigger points cause a shortening of the muscle and refer pain to other areas of the body.

Active trigger points hurt all the time and don't seem to let up; 'latent' trigger points can be an old familiar pain that is triggered by normal movement or daily routine that seem innocent but become active for no apparent reason. Active trigger points are sometimes associated with one or more secondary trigger points which develop when the patient has tried to work it out, strengthen and or stretch the area to get rid of the pain. The surrounding fascia must be released before any attempts to strengthen or stretch it.

This fascia is a never ending continuous membrane that lines the entire body covered with a mucus membrane fluid. This membrane separates the inside of the body from the outside world and provides protection from viruses and other invaders. This membrane much like the skin is composed of elastin and collagen.

Fascia contains nerves and blood vessels that go to the organs in the area that the fascia is found. This fascia tissue provides real-estate or support structure for the vessels and nerves. Blood vessels and nerves travel within the fascia to arrive at their designated end organs. As one could see, when fascia is interrupted, cut, crushed, or damaged in any way the results can affect the body parts that it supports.

CHAPTER 13

The One Hour Massage

You should base the time for a massage on the basis of one hour. If you are doing a basic relaxation massage, you can address most of the muscles in that time. Most people have their schedules based on hour intervals or perhaps have other appointments during the day as well. You need a basis to schedule your appointments and allow enough time to reschedule the next treatment, exchange money, and ample time for the patient to disrobe and dress without feeling rushed.

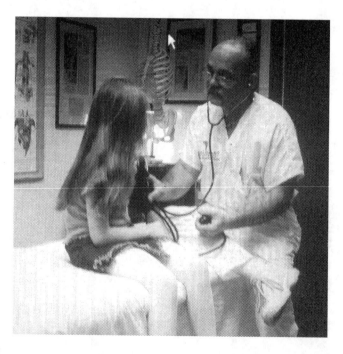

Your treatment room should be designed with relaxation in mind. Tranquil colors without bright lights that shout out at you. If possible use natural daylight. Provide the patient with clothing hooks to place their clothing and valuables like jewelry purse, coat etc. Suggest that they turn off their cell phone so it will not interrupt the session. Show the patient where the restroom is before the session starts and it's a good idea to have access to a sink to wash your hands in front of the patient. Have a blanket ready or on the table if this person has a tendency to be cold. A robe would be convenient if the patient requires a trip to the restroom during the session. Have a box of tissues in your room and a glass of cold water or nearby for a drink if your patient needs it.

Provide some background music to set the mood and provide a relaxing environment for the session. Your choice of music should have a tempo of no more than 60 beats per minute so their sub-conscience does not race and fight against what you are trying to accomplish. Instrumentals are best because some people are reminded of bad experiences by certain songs. Try choosing music with natural backgrounds of nature like the surf ocean, forest, sounds mixed with the soft music. Not too loud. The temperature of the room is important. Usually the patient is disrobed and requires a little more warmth or perhaps the person is elderly and chills easily. Try using some incense to add to your environment.

Before you leave the treatment room you need to instruct your patient how to prepare for their massage, how to lay on the table and inquire if there are any issues they are dealing with that you may help to remove the discomfort or pain. As far as medical history you should have already seen the form they fill out prior to the session for any contra-indications to massage, or conditions like pregnancy or medical conditions to deal with.

Knock softly on the treatment room door to make sure they are ready and enter. Place some massage oil on your hands and apply it to the area you are planning on starting on.

I start with the patient supine, (facing) on their back. I find that starting with the hands is the least invasive to introduce someone to massage as they may not be comfortable with this stranger who is going to give them a rubdown. Perhaps this is their first massage. As you work on the appendages of the body, grip and hold the arms and legs with a firm reassuring hold to transmit a sense of control to the patient. This will make your patient feel that they don't have to help you by holding their arm up and not relaxing it. It transmits a feeling of control and allows the person to relax even more thus helping your work. If you let go of a arm when its perpendicular to the table and it just stays there without dropping the patient is not relaxed.

You will learn very quickly if they want to talk or just experience the quiet and sink into their own thoughts to relax.

The following procedure for an hour massage is what I have been doing for many years. It is based on the suggestion and procedure form the American Medical Association. This massage addresses most of the major muscle groups of the body and designed to relax the patient, and remove stress. When preformed enough times, it will address most problems. After you have more experience you will redesign your program and tune it to suit your needs. You need to zero in on the problem and learn how to remedy it. As you gain more experience and attend more seminars, learn from fellow therapist and add more tools to your therapy toolbox your session will be molded to suite your style.

The most unthreatening body part to start with is the hands. Lubricate the entire right arm starting at the shoulders and spread the oil downward towards the hands. Use a light motion and gentle gliding pressure to spread it uniformly. Gently lift the right hand of the patient with the palm facing up. Support it with your palm of the left hand and the heel of your right hand sandwiching the patients hand pressing firmly with a slight rotation about three times. Rotate the patients hand 180 degrees and repeat the process on the back of the hand. Keep the patients elbow on the table placing both hands around the wrist and slide down to the elbow using your thumb on the forearm and your fingers on the opposite side. When you reach the end of your stroke, repeat the process with the other hand, alternating several times.

Raise the arm and place the wrist under your left arm supported against your side thus freeing your left hand and repeat the process for the upper arm stopping at the patient's armpit. Pay attention to the deltoids, and palpate for sore spots.

Return the arm back to the side of the patient where you initially started and proceed to do friction. This time when you pick up the hand place it palm down and precede to friction each pad of the finger with your index finger proceed down to the last joint one finger at a time. Note that in most cases, arthritis usually starts in the Basal joint. If your patient is older there may be some discomfort. In your female patients, look for Hebrides's Nodes. It is evident when each joint is swollen and range of motion is limited. This form of Osteoarthritis is painful in the finger joints and in time goes away but the large joint stays the same size. Rotate the hand palm with the back of the hand on top of your palm that is supporting it. Friction between your patient's metacarpals with your finger tips in a circular motion while moving upward to the wrist. Rotate the palm up and friction the forearm on both sides. With the patients elbow supported by the table, friction down to it from the wrist and then lift the arm and support it between your arm and side. Use friction on the upper arm ending at the arm pit. If the arm is large and muscular, try a wringing friction. This is done with the arm held up by the wrist. Place both of your hands around the wrist one under the other, grip the tissue with both arms, twist your hands in opposite directions, release both hands while still supporting the arm in a vertical fashion and slide down allowing your hands to re-position in a lower spot on the patients arm and repeat the process again until you reach the end of the arm or the armpit. If you find a hot spot or a spot that needs attention by releasing in the deltoids, bend the hand so that the fingers are pointing or nearly touching the deltoids while the elbow is raised. This position shortens the fibers of the deltoids so that they are not stretched and will release more readily without working against themselves.

Each step of this procedure is repeated 3 times before you change to effleurage or friction, and finally joint movements.

Joint movement is executed next. Joint movement is done to remove the waste product that is deposited after loading the joint with effleurage and friction.

Starting at the fingers you move the end joints while isolating the adjacent one. Proceed to each finger the same way. Grip the fingers and bend them all forward and backward. Grip the hand and bend the entire hand forward and backward, then rotate sideways twisting slightly to both sides. Support the elbow with your palm up while gripping the wrist. Bend the lower arm up to the deltoid and back down. Maintain your grip on the wrist after extending it back to its original location. Isolate the upper forearm with one hand while holding the wrist, rotate the wrist clockwise and counter-clockwise while isolating the elbow. This movement rotates the ulna and radius. After stretching the forearm and all the attached soft tissues, proceed to the shoulder and stretch it by gripping the wrist. Pull the arm keeping it straight and lift the wrist with enough pressure to not allow the elbow to bend in an arc to 180 degrees backwards till it is extended past the head in a parallel to the table. Keep stretching it and return it in the same manner till the wrist is returned to the starting position. Grip the wrist with both hands and stretch the arm again then release it gently. As a finishing touch start at the shoulder and using both hands lightly stroke the arm ending at the finger tips. Do this movement three times progressively lighter and softer. Repeat the entire procedure on the other arm.

Lubricate the upper thoracic area from shoulder to shoulder, including the clavicles and the upper pectorals. Slide across from shoulder to shoulder, then around the outside deltoid and extending across the trapezoids into the Levator scapula upwards to the insertion point. This across the body steady movement is used with a lot of pressure and applied with the flat of your hand. As you go around the deltoid, lock your wrist and pull into the body as you slide into the trapezoids and up the neck. Repeat this from the opposite side of the table.

Standing at the end of the table, behind the patients head, slide your left hand under the back of the head cupping the sub-occipital. Lift and pull at the same time while your left hand slides down the neck and along the trapezoids to the deltoid. You should tilt slightly the head in the opposite direction of the side that you are working. Work the area with your thumb sliding down from the head to the shoulder while looking for sore spots to release.

Starting at the outside of the pictorial and working to the sternum use effleurage and search for sore spots to release. Release with friction of the thumb. Follow the fibers from insertion to origin.

Next in the procedure is the leg. Lubricate from top to foot with long light strokes with the palms of your hands. Start by lifting the knee up into a bent leg position. Reach for the ankle and slide up the back of it alternating by sliding your hand from the ankle to the knee. In the same manner slide from the knee down to the beginning of the leg, repeat on the sides and the back approximately three times each.

Next step is to do friction on the leg. Support the foot with the palm of your hand and do friction with you fingers along the metatarsals beginning at the toes and along the top of the foot in a circular movement. Proceed up the calf and ending at the knee. Do the back of the thigh and then lay the leg down and deep tissue work the quadriceps. After using friction on all of these leg muscles, we need to do the joint movement.

Grab the foot with both hands and rotate it within its range of motion, pronate and supinate and stretch the ankle by pushing the balls of the foot towards the knee. This stretches the Achilles tendon. Place one hand behind the knee and the other support the arch of the foot and push the foot towards the chest until the knee comes close or touches the upper body. Bring the knee back again until the thigh is 90 degrees from the table surface. Keep the let in this position with both hands in place and rotate the thigh in a wide circular fashion to flex the sacroiliac joint and Trochanter joints. Straighten the leg back out and stretch the entire leg by pulling it straight with both hands around the ankle. Pull steady without jerking. Hold the leg for a second or two after the stretch and add a couple of tugs to finish up the joint movement. Repeat again on the other leg.

This brings us to the half way mark in the hour massage which should be close to approximately 30 minutes. Have your patient turn over at this point. They should be given the opportunity to choose between a pillow and a face cradle to support their head.

Start at the low back and apply oil with both hands and spread evenly in long gliding motion. I usually start on the left side of the table and place one hand on top of the other on the left side of the spine base about S1. Lock your elbows and lean into the tissue pushing and gliding upward slowly till you run out of back. Let your weight do the work without pushing with your arms. Position your right leg back with your left knee bent to adjust for height. Do this stroke about 3 times and try to remember the hard spots, the ones that are more dense than the surrounding tissues. You sometimes will notice a spot that is hot or cold. Hot spots are recent injuries, and cold ones are old ones where the blood is going around it rather that addressing it. Make a mental note and spend a little more time on these areas. As you work them you will improve your palpation skills and eventually feel them release under your thumb. Switch sides of the table and repeat it again. As you begin a new technique you can do both sides of the back from one side if you wish but I prefer to switch sides. You can decide which works for you. Next I do a gentle rocking motion to relax the muscles more. You push with your hands in the same position, one on top of the other, push slightly away from the spine and let the body return on its own and gradually move upward repeating the movement. If your patient is elderly or less muscular, try putting your palms together each facing out from the spinal column. Alternate the pressure pushing out and walk your way up with the gentle rocking fashion. Next do long gentle strokes and relax the tissues again. Note that you alternate pressure strokes and then relaxation strokes. Standing at the head of the patient's place both hands on the shoulders and slide down to the iliac crest. Next place your thumbs on each side of the spine and slide down using a circular motion as you move down. Next lay your forearms on the back with hands facing opposite directions and palms down grip the opposite sides. Pull at the same time into the spine with downward pressure. When the palms meet, rotate hands around until fingers meet then slide out to the sides again. Rotate and grab the sides again and repeat back and forth until you arrive at the end of the spine.

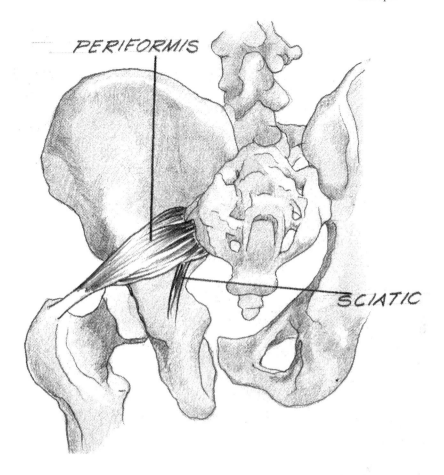

PERIFORMIS

SCIATIC

At this stage, you should check the Sciatica for pain and release it. You can do this by bending the lower leg so the thigh is flat on the table and the lower leg is vertical from the table surface. Bend over slightly and place your elbow on the sciatic nerve where it exits directly under the Periformis is and apply pressure by leaning your body weight slightly and being careful not to overdue the pressure. Hold this position until you feel the

Periformis release.

You will feel your elbow sink slightly as this happens. Depending upon how much the muscle has been abused or traumatized and how long this condition has been going on it may take more than one treatment.

Knee pain:

If this complaint is on the front of the leg I usually find that the quadriceps are strained and the sides of the knee are the result. Massage the quadriceps and stretch them out to release the stress on the knee. The insertion of the quadriceps usually pull on the on the skin of the bone where they attach and make the knee ache. If the complaint is on the behind side of the knee check the popliteal muscle.

This muscle has the distinction of having the longest tendon in the body. The tendon travels down the calf to the arch of the foot and attaches there. There is usually pain in the arch of the foot when this muscle is strain. Treatment is direct trigger point pressure on the belly of the Popliteus muscle for relief.

Apply some oil to the posterior leg starting at the top of the Bicep Femoris and glide down to the foot. Make this movement several to disperse the oil as evenly as you can. Grab the foot by placing one hand under the foot (which would normally be the top) and the other around the balls of the foot. Slide the bottom hand towards the toes using a friction and the upper hand towards the heel. Switch hands and do the same several times.

Next, hold the foot with one hand and use the other hand to glide down the calf of the leg and at the same time move the muscle back and forth sideways in a gliding motion to loosen it up. Place the lower leg back down to the table. Continue to work the upper leg with a strong gliding motion by griping the leg with both hands having your fingers facing opposite directions. Return to the back of the knee and work your way back up the posterior thigh again by griping the muscles with each hand slowly stair stepping upwards stopping at the base of the buttocks. Next, start at the back of the knee again and make a fist with each hand knuckle to knuckle. Together push upwards and rotate your fists in half moon arch's from the middle to the outside of the leg. Finish the leg by starting at the heel and place both hands side by side and glide upwards to the end of the leg flaring out to the sides and spreading your fingers to cover the wider areas several times. Repeat on the other leg.

Ask your patient how they feel, make sure that you have addressed their issues, any questions as to what to expect or if they should need another appointment. Thank them for the visit and ask if they have any needs like a glass of water.

These simple seated stretches are great to do when you've been sitting at your desk for a long time! They will help to reduce stress and re-energize you.

Do them slowly and with control, and don't go to the point of pain.

You deserve to take a few minutes throughout your day to do these seated stretches—your body will thank you for it!

Neck:

Turn your head to the right, then the left. Look up, look down, right ear to shoulder, assist with right hand, left ear to shoulder, assist with left hand.

Shoulder:

Pull your shoulders up, push them down. Round your shoulders forward, press them back. Shoulder circles forward, then backwards.

Arms/Wrists/Hands:

Extend both arms in front of you, palms facing floor. Rotate arms so that palms face up, then back with thumbs down. With your right arm extended in front of you, point fingers towards ceiling, assist the stretch with the left hand. Relax hand, then make fist, and stretch downwards, assisting with other hand. Repeat with left arm/wrist.

Extend both arms out to your side at shoulder height. Make fists again and do wrist circles one direction, then the other.

Stretching is a good way to prolong the hard work you do on your patients and it is a good idea for you to educate your clients how important they are to extend the results of the massage. These procedures will establish a team effort on you and your patient and give them the feeling of something that they can do to maintain control and enhance their life style for a healthier work day when performed at the work place.

Lower Back:

Still sitting in your chair, let your arms hang at your sides, slowly lean over and let your upper body hang downwards. Inhale, then on the exhale let yourself relax further down. Repeat breathing/stretching. Slowly roll back up, one vertebrae at a time, using your arms to assist you if necessary.

Here's another way to stretch your lower back. Sitting upright in your chair, rest your hands palm side down on your desk. Push your chair back until your arms are straight in front of you, while letting your back stretch out so that you are now facing the floor. Take a few deep breaths, and let yourself sink further into the stretch.

Legs/Hips:

Sitting at the edge of your chair, place your hands under your right thigh, and bring that knee up towards your chest. Hold for a few counts, then release. Repeat with the left leg.

Still sitting at the edge of your chair, place your right ankle on your left knee. Bend forward, keeping your back straight, and rest your arms on your legs. Hold for a few counts, then release. Repeat on the other side.

Cross your right ankle over your left knee. Wrap your arms around your right leg and pull your leg in towards your left shoulder. You should feel a slight stretch in your right hip. Stay seated upright while doing this. Repeat with the left leg.

Feet:

Extend out your right leg, point toes upwards, then downwards. Do circles with foot clockwise, then counter-clockwise. Repeat with left leg.

Remember to breathe while doing the stretches!

If possible, get up and walk around the office, or go for a walk on your next break. It not only helps your body, it helps to clear your mind, so that you can approach your work with more clarity.

When you have an athlete, stretching can do a lot for the competitive patient. Take care of your body after you exercise and your body will benefit. It will help your muscles repair themselves and function well during exercise and while at rest. The American College of Sports Medicine recommends doing eight to 10 stretches twice per week. After exercise, the muscles are warm and are malleable— stretch or massage them to increase elongation, flexibility and to prevent delayed onset muscle soreness.

Increased Flexibility

Static stretching (lengthening muscles while they are at rest), and regular massage release muscular tension, returning tight constricted muscles to their normal state of length. Increased flexibility can make activities of daily living such as bending over, standing, squatting or carrying items easier. Improvements in flexibility can improve sports performance. Loosening tight hamstrings can lead to improved speed, endurance and distance for a runner.

Stretching prior to competition can improve circulation, break down lactic acid and release tight muscle for improved performance. When the circulation of blood is enhanced, more oxygen is delivered to the muscle cells and this means more energy. Pre massage and stretching will help the athlete reach the peak performance such as a runner in a shorter amount of time when the athletic activity starts the muscle groups used are at a level with more oxygen. Range of motion is also improved without imbalances less injury, which improves speed, force and balance.

Post massage and stretching will restore the soft tissues to normality by removing lactic acid buildup and lessen recovery time. The traumatized muscle needs to recover from the activity and be cleansed. Stretching will accomplish this along with electrolytes.

CHAPTER 14

How does massage affect our bodies?

The Influence of massage on the therapist's thumb:

Keep in mind that over the years your thumbs take a lot of pressure to perform the many sessions on your patients. This is one of the pitfalls that therapists face and sometimes cut their careers short because of thumb pain. You can use a wooden tool called a "P" ball. This can be held in the palm of your hand to apply pressure instead of your thumb. You can feel the pressure and the muscle release through the tool after a short time of use and preserve the thumbs. It is said that the average career of the therapist is 7 years if body mechanics are not adhered to.

The Influence of massage on the skin:

Massage mechanically cleanses the skin by helping to remove dead epidermis cells. This improves the function of sebaceous and sweats glands. Improvement of the sweat glands improves the extraction of waste through sweating.

The blood vessels dilate and by improving the blood flow the skin is nourished. During energetic effleurage the histamine is extracted from tissues, (particularly the skin) which cause dilation of the vessels. This also increases the temperature of the skin. Massage changes the distribution of the blood by influence of the autonomic nerve of the skin. Massage improves the function of the skins metabolic activity and secreting function.

The Influence of massage on the muscles:

Massage can actually strengthen the muscles with special strokes to simulate contraction and lengthening of muscle fiber during exercise. Elasticity increases and the contraction function with improved electrical activity of the muscle increase. Since the muscle power increases so does the working ability. When petrossage is used, the capillary width increases in the massaged muscle (Kunishev, 1979). The number of open capillaries in normal tissue is approximately 37, after exercise it can be improved to 3700. Since more blood is needed while performing exercise, and massage decreasing the lactic acid and other organic acids, allowing room for more oxygen. Acid buildup in tissue restricts the amount of oxygen intake ability. This is why atrophy is reduced in striated and smooth muscle tissues when massage is applied.

The influence of massage on the ligaments tendons and joints:

Elasticity and flexibility in the tendinous connections and joints are enhanced from massage and stretching. As a result, injuries are fewer which used to be a common reason for problems in the joints is. The release of synovial fluid and increase production after massage lubricate the joints and tendons. Deep tissue work helps to remove waste buildup, fluids, and edema to restore better range of motion. The rehabilitation of joints benefit more from this than any other technique. Heat, generated by friction massage can sustain remissions in such dysfunctions as arthritis because of the increased blood flow and heat.

Influence of massage on the cardiovascular system:

One of the most important functions of massage is to move blood. When massage is applied, movement of the blood flows through the whole body from the organs to the skin and muscle tissues causes the peripheral vessels to start to increase moderately. In turn the heart works less because the left ventricle eases and the blood supply is enhanced. The efficiency of contractibility of the heart muscle increases. More capillaries are opened which increases the amount of oxygen available to the tissues. The local temperature of the massaged area increases from ½ degree to 3 degrees

C. The blood circulates 9 to 140 times better. Blood pressure decreases (systolic 5 to 15 mm, diastolic 5 to 10mm). (Kurashova Kurashova Wine 1984) If you keep track of the BP before and after massage even sometimes as much as the next day, massage can be used to train the cardiovascular system. Assisting the flow of blood and enhancing the circulatory system can increase oxygen absorption and feeding the cells of tissue improve. The quality of blood is improved through massage by increased hemotogenic function. by adding hemoglobin and erythrocytes. The immune system benefits because leukocytes are increased in the blood.

Influence of massage on the nervous system:

Massage can slow the nervous system down or speed it up depending on the goals of the therapist. Effleurage brings positive emotions to a relaxation state. Vibration and petrossage excites and stimulate the nervous system. The nervous system is the controlling switch panel for the body systems by regulation of the size or dilation of vessels. It increases the expansion of capillaries and the exchange of blood between tissues. Massage can control the sympathetic nervous system to some degree, and enhance the peripheral nervous system for help with recovery in surgery or injuries.

Influence of massage on the lymph flow:

Massage improves the lymphatic flow up to 8 times. By assisting in the removal of waste from the cells, the nourishment of the cells and tissues free the cells from the products of metabolism (metabolites and catabolism).

Influence of massage on the respiratory system:

By stretching the muscles of the repertory function, it increases deep inhalation and exhalation. Massage of the lower part of the rib cage will increase ventilation and blood circulation in the lower part of the lungs. Massage of chest and back will normalize the rhythm of breathing, of the repercussion such as cupping helps the removal of mucus, and the lungs and restores elasticity.

CHAPTER 15

Advanced Muscle Release Procedures

The following is an account of re-occurring problems that I have been exposed to over the years with my patients. I felt that the treatments for these merit mentioning. General massage will address most injuries when done enough times. There is a definite advantage of diagnosing muscle problems and getting results by the end of the treatment session without a lot of return visits.

Fingers tingling and numb:

This is usually a sign of brachial plexus impingement.

There are five nerves that are born from the spinal column between the scapula and spine. These nerves exit this area and wrap around the rotator cuff and ultimately end in the tips of each of the five fingers of the same arm. Muscle trauma and injury edema applies pressure to these nerves causing them to ache, feel like pins and needles, and go numb. The scalene muscles on the same side of the neck along with the trapezoids, and Levator Scapula contribute to this condition. Work on these muscle groups using deep techniques along with stretching, and stokes that relax to restore the muscles to normal tension. Any time something swells means that something has to compress. There are no voids in the body and no room for expansion. Something has to give way, in this case it is the nerves. Sometimes this condition is misdiagnosed as Carpal Tunnel Syndrome.

This condition is very often misdiagnosed as carpal tunnel syndrome. To verify this, there is a test that can tell you if the brachial plexus is impinged. Have your patient turn the palm of the affected arm palm up. Bend the fingers to touch the tips of the fingers and the base of the fingers on the last pad before the fingers start. If your patient cannot do this and touches the palm because they cannot bend the fingers enough but further down the palm close to the thumb instead. After this movement raise the arm up and place the hand behind the head and try this movement again. If the patient succeeds by touching the right place on the palm it means the brachial plexus is pinched.

Shoulder/Deltoid pain:

The shoulder/deltoid muscle is divided into three sections. The Anterior deltoid raises your arm forward and up. The lateral deltoid raises your arm out sideways and the posterior deltoid lifts the arm towards the rear and up. Depending on the complaint of your patient, determine which section of the shoulder is damaged by the motion that is difficult to perform. Treatment release is while the patient is supine on the table, bend the arm until the hand can be laid upon the deltoid of the same arm, then raise the elbow up almost vertical. This position shortens the fibers in the deltoid without stretching it out so when friction or pressure is applied to the fibers they will release easier because they are not stretched out and working against them.

Trapezoids pain

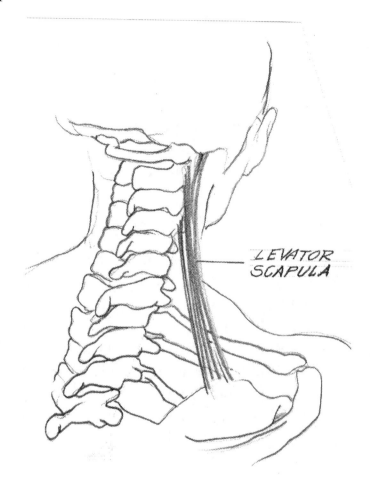

LEVATOR SCAPULA

Treatment for tight painful muscle fibers in the Trapezius can be released by having the patient sit in a straight back chair with spine erect. Have your patient relax the arm of the side being treated so it is placid and hanging. Place your forearm across the Trapezius with your hand on the wrist of the arm using the forearm. Have your patient totally relax as you press down with your forearm stretching the Trapezius and lean your body weight into it in a downward direction. Hold this for about 10 to 15 seconds and release slowly. At this point instruct your patient to resist by pushing up against your forearm and try to match with equal pressure. Hold this position for about 10 seconds. Instruct your patient to relax as you do the same by releasing your pressure at the same time.

Next stretch it out by pressing and stretching as you did in the first step. Push down and hold this position for about 10 seconds. This procedure is very good to relax the Levator Scapula in the same way.

This muscle contributes greatly to most headache complaints. Part of the insertion to the sub-occipital ridge is the key. When the muscle is traumatized, it shortens and pulls on the Pariosteum or the skin of the bone and the Occipitalis muscle. The occipital muscle contracts which tightens the Ape neurosis which is like a wide flat tendon and connects to the Frontalis muscle, and thus tightens. This whole procedure causes tightness and pressure on the skull and becomes a headache.

TMJ Dysfunction:

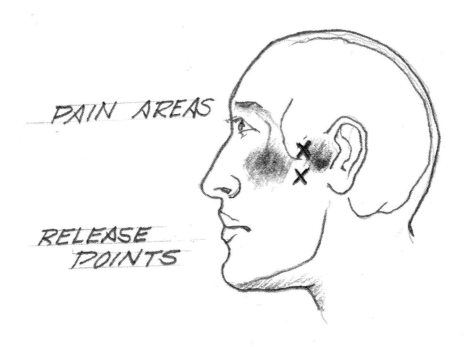

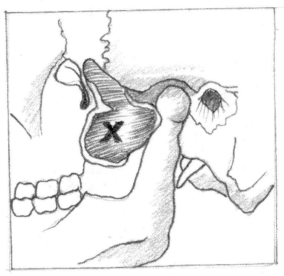

The Pterygoid lateral can release a lot of discomfort caused by TMJ dysfunction. If the pain of the mandibular joint is on the left side, use a finger cot to cover your index finger of the left hand and palpate the Pterygoid from the inside. Push with gentle pressure on it and at the same time use your right index finger to press on the outside to trap the muscle an feel the release. This procedure can reduce suffering for a person who suffers from TMJ. It will not correct the situation but is a temporary fix. Eventually the mandible muscle will pull enough when you chew, your jaw articulates with the skull enough times it will widen the hole that it goes through. There is a disc on the inside of the skull that this muscle anchors to and the disc will wear down to the point that it pull through the opening. This is the popping sound you hear when you chew. Left unchecked it will worsen to the point that the muscle will pull a nerve bank located past the disc through the hole to the point that when you chew it is very painful. Your dentist can supply a bite plate to keep you from grinding your teeth and re-align the jaw. Corrective surgery can remedy this in advanced cases. The use of moist heat placed on the pain area surface will help relieve the discomfort. Advise your patient not to chew gum on occasion this condition will improve with the removal of stress in the patient's life.

TMJ RELEASE

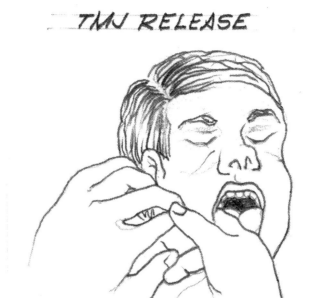

You will find some situations where you cannot insert your finger into the patient mouth because it will not open enough to accommodate the finger width. In any case the use of finger cots will be necessary to protect the patient and preserve a sanitation environment. Once you release this muscle there is a marked change in the pain level and several days to weeks of relief may be expected. If you can remove the reason for the misalignment of the mandible in relationship to the upper skull, with bite plates designed by a dentist and notice the relief of pain lasting longer after each treatment you may expect recovery.

Strain/Counter Strain:

One of the most effective methods of releasing a painful muscle is Strain Counter/strain technique. This was discovered by Dr. Lawrence Jones DO. Some have referred to it as positional release, the Levitt stretching release, passive positional release and the list goes on. The patient assists in the procedure. After discovering the trigger point and the muscle/muscles involved, you need to determine if it is an adductor or abductor, or extensor rather than a flexor. Then you can decide which movement puts the muscle in the resting position. Leave your hand on the trigger point and palpate when the pain level is less and the pain experienced by the patient is the most comfortable. Hold this position for 90 seconds. This time period seems to be the magic number and occasionally it may take as long as a few more minutes. Gently tighten the muscle afterwards and attempt to move it in the full range of motion. The pain is usually much less. If this release stays and reduces the discomfort after a day or two, try moving the muscle to the new point of contraction with the patient trying to contract the muscle and you resist the movement further. Hold this position for about 2 or 3 seconds and have the patient release the contraction. This is called applied muscle energy, or the counter/strain of the technique. Try this about 6 times or more and observe the extension and new restored range of motion.

CHAPTER 16

Trigger point areas suggested:

The following is a list of possible pain or trigger point areas and the associated soft tissues that may be involved.

Head and Neck pain

Back of Head: Trapezius, Sternocleidomastoid both sternal and clavicular

Front of Head: Sternocleidomastoid, Semispinalis capitis, Frontalis, Zygomaticus Major

Ear & TMJ Pain: Lateral Pterygoid, Masseter deep, Sternocleidomastoid, Medial Pterygoid,

Throat & Front of Neck Pain: Sternocleidomastoid, Digastric, Medial Pterygoid

Back of Neck Pain: Trapezius, Multifidi, Levator Scapulae, Splenius cervicis, Infrapinatus.

Temporal Headache: Trapezius, Sternocleidomastoid, Temporalis, Splenius Cevicis, Suboccipital Group, Semispinalis capitis.

Back Of Head Pain: Sternocleidomastoid, Semispinalis capitis, Semispinalis cervicis, Suboccipital group, Occipitalis, Digastric, Temporalis

Vertex Pain, (top of head): Sternocleidomastoid.

Cheek & Jaw Pain: Sternocleidomastoid, Masseter, Lateral Pterygoid, Trapezius, Masseter, Digastric, Medial Pterygoid, Buccinator, Platyma, Orbicularis Ocular, Zygomaticus Major.

Toothache: Temporalis, Masseter, Digastric.

Upper Thoracic Back Pain: Scaleni, Levator Scapulae, Supraspinatus, Trapezius, Multifidi, Rhomboidei, Splenius Cervicis, Triceps Brachii, Biceps Brachii

Mid-Thoracic Back Pain: Scaleni, Latissimus Dorsi, Levator Scapulae, Iliocostalis Thoracis, Multifidi, Rhomboidei, Serratus Posterior Superior, Infrapinatus, Trapezius, Serratus Anterior.

Back of Shoulder Pain: Deltoid, Levator Scapulae, Supraspinatus, Teres Major, Teres Minor, Subscapularis, Serratu Posterior Superior, Latissimus Dorsi, Triceps Brachii, Trapezius, Iliocostalis Thoracis,

Back of Arm Pain: Scaleni, Triceps Brachii, Deltoid, Subscapularis, Supraspinatus, Teres Major, Teres Minor, Latissimus Dorsi, Serratus Posterior Superior, Coracobrachialis, Scalenus Minimus

Low Thoracic Back Pain: Iliocostalis Thoracis, Multifidi, Serratus Posterior Inferior, Rectus Abdominis, Intercostals, Latissimus Dorsi, Iliopsoas,

Lumbar Pain: Longissimus Thoracis, Iliocostalis Lumborum, Iliocostalis Thoracis, Multifidi, Rectus Abdominis.

Sacral & Gluteal Pain: Longissimus Thoracis, Iliocostalis Lumborum, Multifidi.

Front of Chest Pain: Pectoralis Major, Pectoralis Minor, Scaleni, Sternocleidomastoid, Sternalis, Intercostals, Iliocostalis Cervicis, Subclavius, Abdominal Oblique, Diaphragm.

Abdominal Pain: Rectus Abdominis, Abdominal Obliques, Transverus Abdominis, Iliocostalis Thoracis, Multifidi, Pyramidalis, Quadratus Lumborum.

Lumbar Pain: Iliopsoas, Gluteus Medias, Periformis.

Sacral & Gluteal Pain: Quadratus Lumborum, Periformis, Gluteus Medius, Gluteus Maximus, Levator Ani, Coccygeus, Soleus.

Side of Chest Pain: Serratus Anterior, Intercostals, Latissimus Dorsi, Diaphragm.

Abdominal Pain: Rectus Abdominis, Obliquus Externus Abdominis, Thoracis, Multifidi, Quadratus Lumborum, Pyramidalis,

Lumbar Pain: Gluteus Medius, Multifidi, Iliopsoas, Longissimus Thoracis, Rectus Abdominis, Iliocostalis Thoracis, Iliocostalis Lumborum.

Buttock Pain: Gluteus Medius, Quadratus Lumborum, Gluteus Maximus, Iliocostalis Lumborum, Longissimus Thoracis, Semitendinosus & Semimembranosus, Periformis, Gluteus Minimus, Rectus Abdominis, Soleus.

S I Joint Pain/Iliosacral Pain: Levator Ani & Coccygeus, Gluteus Medius, Quadratus Lumborum, Gluteus Maximus, Multifidi, Iliopsoas, Longissimus Thoracis, Rectus Abdominis, Iliocostalis Thoracis, Iliocostalis Lumborum.

Pelvic Pain: Obturator Infernus, Coccygeus, Levator Ani, Adductor Magnus, Periformis, Obliquus Internus Abdominis.

Anterior Knee Pain: Rectus Femoris, Vastus Medialis, Adductors Longus & Brevis,

Anterior Thigh Pain: Adductors Longus & Brevis, Iliopsoas, Adductor Magnus, Vastus Intermedius, Pectineus, Sartorius, Quadratus Lumborum, Rectus Femoris.

Lateral Knee Pain: Vastus Lateralis,

Lateral Knee & Hip Pain: Gluteus Maximus, Gluteus Minimus, Vastus Lateralis, Periformis, Quadratus Lumborum, Tensor Fasciae Late, Vastus Intermedius, Vastus Lateralis, Rectus Femoris.

Medial Thigh Pain: Pectineus, Vastus Medialis, Cracilis, Adductor Magnus, Sartorius.

Posterior Knee Pain: Gastrocnemius, Biceps Femoris, Popliteus, Semitendinosis & Semimembranosus, Soleus, Plantaris.

Posterior Thigh Pain: Gluteus Minimus, Semimembranosus & Semitendinosus, Bicepts Femoris, Periformis, Obturator Internus.

Anterior Ankle Pain: Tibialis Anterior, Peroneus Tertius, Extensor Digiitorum Longus, Extensor Hallucis Longus.

Anterior Leg Pain: Tibialis Anterior, Adductors Longus Brevis.

Great Toe Pain (Bottom): Tibialis Anterior, Extensor Hallucis Longus, Extensor Hallucis Brevis.

Forefoot Pain, (Bottom): Extensor Digitorum Brevis, Extensor Hallucis Brevis, Extensor Digitorum Longus, Extensor Hallucis Longus, Extensor Hallucis Brevis, Interossei of foot, Tibialis Anterior.

Heel Pain: Soleus, Quadratus Planate, Abductor Hallucis, Tibialis Posterior.

Lateral Ankle Pain: Peronei Longus & Brevis, Peroneus Tertius

Lateral Leg Pain: Gastrocnemius, Gluteus Minimus anterior section, Peronei Longus & Brevis, Vastus Lateralis.

Medial Ankle Pain: Abductor Hallucis, Flexor Digitorum Longus.

Metatarsal Head Pain: Flexor Hallucis Brevis, Digitorum Brevis, Abductor Hallucis, Extensor Hallucis Longus, Interossei of foot, Flexor Hallucis Brevis, Tibialis Posterior,

Great Toe Pain (bottom): Flexor Hallucis Longus.

Lesser Toe Pain (bottom): Flexor Digitorum Longus, Tibialis Posterior.

Mid foot Bottom Pain: Gastrocnemius, Flexor Digitorum Longus, Abductor Hallucis, Interossei of Foot, Abductor Hallucis, Tibialis Posterior.

Posterior Ankle Pain: Soleus, Tibialis Posterior.

Posterior Leg Pain: Soleus, Gluteus Minimus, Gastrocnemius, Semitendinosus & Semimembranosus, Flexor Digitorum Longus, Tibialis Posterior, Plantaris.

Sinus congestion:

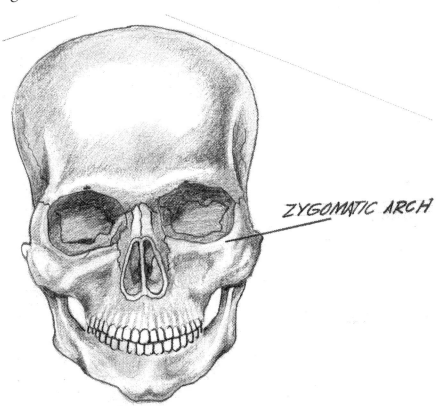

ZYGOMATIC ARCH

To relieve sinus pressure causing headaches, place the patient supine on your table and seat yourself at the end of the table behind the head. When working on the right side of the face, place your right hand with the finger tips resting on the zygomatic arch end near the nose. Place your left hand on the right side f the nasal septum near the nose. Press down with pressure and pull your fingers apart with a slow firmness. This movement opens the crack between the two bones and helps to allow atmospheric pressure to equalize internal pressure. This allows the fluid to drain both internally and externally. A noticeable improvement in breathing through the nose is apparent.

In addition to the above technique, a facial massage with some eucalyptus in your oil or similar additive aids greatly. Apply gentle pressure around the temporal lobes of both sides.

Temporal pain:

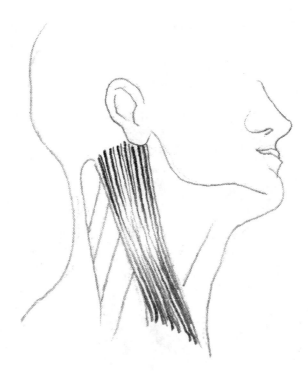

Pain along the side of the forehead can be caused by the (Sternocleidomastoid).

Have the patient supine while you are seated at the head or end of the table. If the discomfort is on the right side of the head, ask the patient to lift their head slightly. This movement flexes the SCM. Grasp the belly of the SCM with your thumb and forefinger. Ask the patient to turn their head slightly to the right. This movement pulls the Ceratoid Artery away so that it cannot be picked up with the SCM. Straighten the head and slight apply pressure until you feel it release. Usually the pain goes away almost immediately.

The SCM (Sternocleidomastoid) Muscle inserts into the upper chest. It splits into a upside down "V" shape and assists in forced inspiration as in taking a deep breath. This is a good muscle to treat when you deal with athletes. Increased breathing capacity will improve repertory performance.

Increased air intake:

By expanding the rib cage the volume of air can be increased after this stretch. With the patient seated on the table, stand behind them and place your knee in the middle of the back. Place your hands in front of the shoulders on the pictorials. Instruct your patient to drop and lower the shoulders and tilt the head forward and down. Take a huge breath, and let it out slowly as the head tilts backward pull the shoulders back at the same time while pressing with your knee. Increased volume is the result. I have used this method on swimmers and vocalist with noted improvement. The intercostals are stretched allowing movement of the ribs with greater range of motion. As much as 30% increase.

CHAPTER 17

Psoas strain:

I would say that this is one muscle that is responsible for most back pain complaints. This technique will prove to be invaluable to you during your practice. Evidence of psoas strain is the complaint of pain on either side of the spine or both sides in an area starting at the iliac crest extending upwards to L5. This muscle lays on top of the transverse processes and cannot be accessed from the posterior. The muscle must be addressed from the front. When traumatized, the pressure on the nerves is caused by expansion of the muscle pressing on the nerve banks trapping them against the transverse processes. Typically the patient is bent slightly forward when standing and sleeps on the side with the knees bent to relieve the discomfort.

Have your patient lay in the supine position with the knees bent to shorten the psoas muscles. When treating the right psoas, place your right hand on the knee, and the left hand with the finger tips pointing down to the stomach. Apply pressure with a small diameter circular motion. This movement will force the colon out of the way to access the muscle. Have your patient lift the foot off of the table in order to flex the muscle in order to identify it. You will feel it flex and become hard. Palpate for the worst spot on it. Press and wait for your hand to sink deeper when it relaxes somewhat. Wait while applying steady pressure and it will dr op down again. The patient will note the referral pain subside in the back at the same time. In some situations, the insertion of the psoas muscle at the top of the femur will be very tender and need releasing also. As this tendon relaxes, you will notice that the knee will slowly drop to the side allow range of motion improvement. While you apply your pressure on the psoas muscle to release it, move the knee to the outside of the body and this will rotate the muscle in such a way that the inside of the muscle presents itself to palpate, then move the knee to opposite side to present the outside for examination.

On the left psoas, caution must be used as this is where the great internal and external iliac veins will be palpated. A judgment call is needed here. When pressure is applied some plaque may release and cause an embolism. If your patient is elderly, or in apparently bad physical condition you should refrain of use less pressure on this psoas.

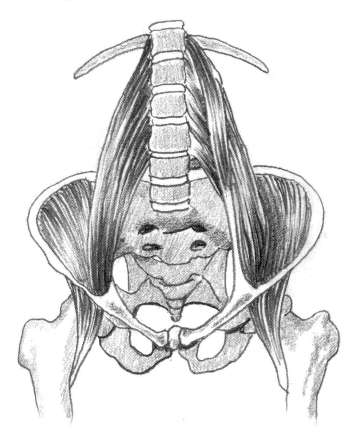

After releasing this muscle you will need to stretch it. Have your patient slide down to the end of the table to the point where it feels like there tailbone is at the edge of the table. Bend the leg of the side of the body that you are not working on and let the leg from the side you are working on hand over the end of the table. Push the bent knee toward the upper body while pushing down with the knee of the other leg. Have your patient push back with this knee at the same time. Have them stop pushing and gently push the knee down a little closer to the floor. Repeat this on the other leg. Done correctly, the patient will experience relief instantaneously after standing.

Sciatica pain:

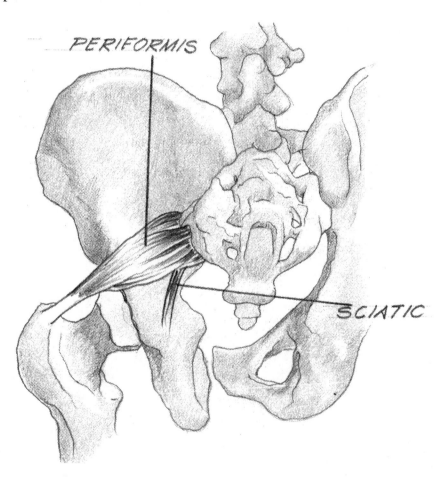

This nerve is quite large, the size of your thumb. The pain is caused usually from the Periformis muscle pressing on it from being traumatized from an accident or heavy lifting. To locate the trigger point, draw an imaginary line from the side of the sacrum to the outer trochanter. In the middle of the line is where you can apply pressure on the belly of the Periformis to release the pain. This nerve ends in the great toe. The pain will diminish as it heals and move back up the thigh to the original orientation in the hip. Apply pressure to the muscle pressing with your elbow gently and note that the elbow will sink slowly down when the release happens.

Knee pain:

If this complaint is on the front of the leg I usually find that the quadriceps is strained and the sides of the knee are the result. Massage the quadriceps and stretch them out to release the stress on the knee. The insertion of the quadriceps usually pull on the on the skin of the bone where they attach and make the knee ache. If the complaint is on the behind side of the knee check the popliteal muscle.

This muscle has the distinction of having the longest tendon in the body. The tendon travels down the calf to the arch of the foot and attaches there. There is usually pain in the arch of the foot when this muscle is strain. Treatment is direct trigger point pressure on the belly of the popliteal muscle for relief.

CHAPTER 18

Resistive Stretching:

Muscle mobility can be restored by using pulling and stretching the muscle fibers while the patient is resisting slightly. For example when the Trapezoid is tight and painful, have the patient sit in a chair with the spine straight. Position yourself standing by the side of the muscle being treated, place your forearm across the top of the trapezoid, and grasp your wrist with the other hand. Bend and lean to push with a force downward with a slow deliberate movement. Hold this position a few seconds and then ask the patient to resist with a push back in the opposite direction you are pushing. Try to match the pressure the patient is using with equal force. Hold this pressure for a few seconds. Have the patient relax and then push down again to stretch it without the patient pushing back.

Occipital Release Resistive Stretch:

Perform this maneuver from a seated position behind or at the end of the table. Your patient is supine. Have your patient move towards you so that the head is past the edge of the table enough to place your hands knuckles down with your fingers together and bent at the first joint making contact at the sub-occipital. Instruct your patient to relax and let the weight of the head sink down onto the fingers. If the patient relaxes enough, the head will gently drop backwards slowly. After the head drops, place your hand around the chin and the other one around the back of the head and pull with both hands gently. Cross your forearms with your palms on each shoulder and the head supported on the forearms. Bend your arms by raising them and your palms remaining on the shoulders. This movement will raise the head to the point of the chin touching the chest. Stop when resistance is experienced and hold it for a few seconds. Have your patient press back and hold this pressure while you attempt to match the same pressure. Hold for a few seconds. Release all forces and pressure. Stretch the head forward again till resistance is met and repeat again. Cradle the head with both hands and rotate in small circles and bend side to side to demonstrate the improvement of the range of motion. Have your patient slide back onto the table so you can place the head down and be supported. Place each hand on the shoulders and alternately push each shoulder towards the feet while stair-stepping up the trapezoids till you reach the neck.

Psoas Release Resistive Stretch:

After treating the psoas as described earlier in this book it will need to be stretched. This treatment last much longer after stretching it. Have your patient lay supine on the table. The positioning of the patient should be such that the coccyx is on the edge of the table. Bend the foot of the side not being treated and place it on your belly. Let the other leg hand down over the table. Gently push down on the knee of the side being treated until resistance is noted. Hold it for a few seconds, and ask the patient to push back against your hand while you match the pressure. Hold for a few seconds, release and gently press the leg down while it is relaxed, hold for a few seconds.

Levator Scapula/ Trapezoid Resistive Stretch:

While your patient is seated in a straight back chair stand at the side and place your forearm across the trapezoid with your other hand gripping your wrist for better support an balance. Lean into and down to stretch it. Instruct your patient to relax and not push back while you do this. Release your pressure and do the same thing but have your patient push back while you try to match their pressure. Hold this position for a few seconds and release the pressure. Have your patient rotate and roll the shoulders to see if the release worked.

These procedures are just a few of the examples of resistive stretch technique. This basic principle will work on just about all your range of motion restoration attempts. By applying these principles you are stretching out the fascia, scar tissues, and re-educating the neuron-transmitters to reset and hold the memory of the muscle in a more relaxed state.

CHAPTER 19

Reflexology:

I use Reflexology to diagnose problems and go directly to the area in distress located on the body. By examining the areas on the feet you will find painful spots and usually a hard knot when you palpate it. I work it with my thumb until it dissipates You are also making changes and corrections by working on the reflex area in the foot to achieve the balance and healing. There are nerves that carry messages to the brain, (afferent), and nerves that carry messages from the brain (efferent). These nerves change from one or the other and travel to the feet then back to the brain. If they are blocked, this technique restores continuity in the electric impulse for the complete message and allows s the body part reflected to restore functionality. It is a complementary therapy, used in conjunction with traditional forms of medical care. Reflexology involves the stimulation of nerves on the feet, hands and ears. Stimulation of nerves on the feet is the primary focus of reflexology. The hands and the ears are most often the site of reflexology treatments when physical constraints (contraindications), such as fractures, are apparent.

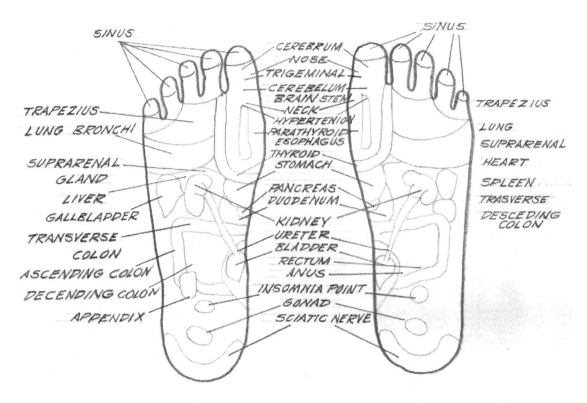

Stimulation of selected locations on the feet, hands, and ears is thought to produce beneficial effects in other parts of the body and to enhance the overall quality of health. There is no one fixed theory to explain reflexology. All practitioners believe that areas on the foot correspond to areas of the body, and that reflexology assists the self-healing process. Some practitioners believe these zones to reflect the energy of the body, and that blockages of energy in the body are reflected through "grit" or "lumps" on the foot.

Iridology:

Another form of reflexology is iridology: I use this method to explain a lot of discomfort my patient reports to me. This method is a good vehicle to predict problems that have not manifested or surfaced to be recognized. You can keep track of the condition and healing process with iridology. Consider using this diagnostic tool to help determine problems and assist your patient in their journey to good health.

Many physicians used this method to diagnose their patient before the advent of the computer. This valuable tool has fallen between the cracks of the examination room floor because of the many new blood tests and other methods that have taken it's place. The iris is the end of the optic nerve consisting of millions of nerve endings. These nerve endings have their origin from all the parts of the body and are a direct extension of each body part. By observation of these areas a reflex ion of the condition of the health of the corresponding body part can be determined. You can track the healing progress by monitoring this part of the iris. Iridology is the analysis of the iris, which is the colorful area of the eye that surrounds the pupil. By analyzing the iris, a person's level of health and specific areas of nutritional deficiency can be identified. This allows appropriate remedies to be recommended.

Iridology is a method to analyze the body's current condition by diagnosing tissue weakness like a throat culture, sphygmomanometer (blood pressure cuff), thermometer, or other tests to reveal the current health condition of the body. This method can also warn you of weaknesses that will manifest themselves into more serious issues down the road than may be avoided. One can verify the cleansing and healing with regular examinations. After observing these problems you can determine a plan of nutrition or treatment to improve the health.

CHAPTER 20

Hyperbaric Oxygen Chamber:

If you have access to a facility with a chamber, it would be helpful to familiarize yourself with this healing tool. Some of the famous sports professional own their own chamber to sleep in during the night to heal from the grueling injuries sustained from combat in the professional football and basketball careers. These chambers can help slow down cancer and in some cases heal it. It is accomplished by contained air pressure about 2 times greater than the atmospheric pressure of the room it is housed in. Higher oxygen content is inside the area the patient is housed in and breathed into the lungs. Oxygen speeds up the healing from the inside out. Wounds heal more quickly with the extra oxygen carried by the blood to infected wounds and the tissues and organs of the body. Bone infections, burn victims, carbon monoxide poisoning, decompression sickness, gangrene, skin graphs, ulcers, and other chronic conditions are very successful with this modality. Usually a treatment is at least an hour or more over the course of several treatments through the week.

Ultrasound and Electrical Stimulus are two treatment modalities that may benefit your practice and offer more healing avenues that you should consider. Your scope of practice may include these forms of treatment and you should check to make sure they are included

Ultrasound:

Ultrasound therapy uses high-energy sound waves (those above the range we hear) to help ease painful joints and muscles. Ultrasound treatment is done by a physical therapist or occupational therapist who guides the waves into the body from the head of a ultrasound machine. Results of using this method for arthritis pain relief will vary.

The use of ultrasonic's to treat disorders such as deep, soft tissue injuries. Ultrasound treatment is believed to have a mechanical effect, accelerating the healing process. vibrating and loosening scar tissue, and encouraging the re-absorption of blood and lymph that has escaped into surrounding tissue. The vibrations may reduce sensory stimulation and relieve pain; they also produce heat at a deep level. Therapeutic ultrasound as a treatment modality has been used by therapists over the last 50 years to treat soft tissue injuries. Ultrasonic waves (sound waves of a high frequency) are produced by means of mechanical vibration of the metal treatment head of the ultrasound machine. This treatment head is then moved over the surface of the skin in the region of the injury. When sound waves come into contact with air it causes a dissipation of the waves, and so a special ultrasound gel is placed on the skin to ensure maximal contact between the treatment head and the surface of the skin.

Ultrasound is one of the best forms of heat treatment for soft tissue injuries. It is used to treat joint and muscle sprains, bursitis, and tendonitis.

Ultrasound treatment is used to:

- relieve pain and inflammation
- speed healing
- reduce muscle spasms and
- increase range of motion

Ultrasound makes high frequency sound waves. The sound waves vibrate tissues deep inside the injured area. This creates heat that draws more blood into the tissues. The tissues then respond to healing nutrients brought in by the blood and the repair process begins.

Treatment is given with a sound head that is moved gently in strokes or circles over the injured area. It lasts just a few minutes. The procedure may be performed with the sound head alone or combined with a topical anti-inflammatory drug or gel.

Ultrasound treatment is often used by physical therapists, trainers, and many other healthcare providers. It is very safe and is never used around the eyes, ears, ovaries, testicles, or spinal cord, or where there is an active infection.

Electrical Stimulus:

Electrical stimulation uses an electrical current to cause a single muscle or a group of muscles to contract. By placing electrodes on the skin in various locations the physical therapist can recruit the appropriate muscle fibers. Contracting the muscle via electrical stimulation helps strengthen the affected muscle. The physical therapist can change the current setting to allow for a forceful or gentle muscle contraction. Along with increasing muscle strength, the contraction of the muscle also promotes blood supply to the area that assists in healing. Electric muscle stimulation (EMS) is touted as having the ability to strengthen muscles, reduce weight, minimize body fat and improve local blood circulation. During physical activity, your brain (inside source) sends a message to nerves to signal the contraction of certain muscles. EMS uses an outside electrical source to communicate with nerve fibers. When the stimulation is applied, the brain sends a nerve impulse to the motor point of the muscle. This signal causes the muscle to expand and contract. EMS sends minute quantities of electricity to the body. Electrodes are placed over the motor points of the muscle group to be exercised. Electrical current is emitted through rubber contact pads that are positioned over particular muscles that tighten when they become aroused by electrical energy. The stimulation is not constant but turns on and off to imitate traditional exercise. This prompts the muscle to passively exercise.

EMS is distinguished by its low volt stimulation that's intended to arouse motor nerves to cause a muscle contraction. Electrical muscle stimulation signals the brain to sends a nerve impulse to the motor point of your muscle.

Sphygmomanometer:

A must have in your treatment room. This device is used to measure blood pressure usually in the vein. Checking your patient is done by wrapping the cuff around the arm above the elbow with the arrow pointing towards the artery just below the bicep. Position the arm so it is resting on a solid surface with the arm slightly bent so the lower arm is parallel to the heart. Make the cuff snug but not too tight by adjusting the sleeve by pulling and adhering the Velcro in position. Place the stethoscope ear pieces into your ears. Place the wide disc of the stethoscope onto the arm just above the elbow just below the bicep on the inside of the arm. The proper position is sometimes easier to find if you place two fingers on the skin an feel the pulse. Turn the valve at the bulb in a clockwise direction to shut it off. Squeeze the bulb in a steady repeated fashion until the gauge indicates about 180. Gently turn the valve on the bulb counter-clockwise to start releasing the pressure in a slow release. As the needle falls listen for the thumping sound and take note of the reading for the first thumping sound. The first thumping sound is the Systolic number of the blood pressure. This is the amount of pressure on the walls of the heart when it compresses and pushes the blood. The bottom number of the blood pressure is when you stop hearing the thumping sound which represents the diastolic or bottom number representing the pressure at heart rest between beats. Note that sometimes it is a good idea to check both arms and see if there is a noted difference between the two readings. If there is a significant higher reading it could be a sign of blocked artery in the neck.

CHAPTER 21

Checking Leg Length:

Are your legs uneven? Leg-length discrepancies are rarely the result of having one leg bone that's truly longer than the other. More often than not, they're caused by a tight hamstring or Iliotibial band that jacks up the other side of the pelvis. Runners with this imbalance tend to overcompensate by favoring their "longer" leg, which can lead to injury. Could this be happening to you? Take this test to find out.

1) Lie on your back, on a flat surface with your legs together, feet bare. Have a friend place the palms of his hands on your hipbones, one hand on the left and one hand on the right.
2) Ask your friend to gently rock your hips back and forth, pressing left, right, left, right, until you are relaxed (about a minute).
3) Now have your friend look at your feet to see if your anklebones are even.

A lot of low back pain can be the result of having a leg shorter than the other Sometimes an injury or surgery may be the reason. Hip replacements, knee surgery or they may have been born that way. The upper torso needs to compensate similar to stacking a pile of books that need to lean to one side or the other to keep the center of gravity changes as weight is transferred to one side of the body. You can see evidence of uneven shoe wear revealing a worn heal or low areas that are not the same on both shoes. Usually either the foot, ankle, knee and hip will be under more stress showing chronic pain, and there will eventually be changes that equalize, that take place above the pelvis as the balance of the spine is changed. Scoliosis may develop with visual discrepancies then joint degeneration on one side of the spine.

There are two types of short leg syndromes and we need to determine which one applies to your patient in order to treat it.

1. Anatomical Short Leg. The measurement from the bony protuberance (the greater trochanter) of the hip joint to the lateral ankle measures shorter on one side than the other. This is seen in approximately three percent of all short-leg syndromes because they were born this way.

2. Functional Short Leg. The measurement from the same two points is equal on both sides, but there is still an apparent short leg. With this type, there is usually a rotation or displacement of the pelvis on one side. This results in stress on all the muscles connected to the pubic and iliac bones including the sacrum, nerves and joints that are involved. The longer a person has this type of short-leg syndrome, obviously the more time the body has to compensate for the difference of the other side. Usually in the upper back, shoulders or neck need to balance by leaning the opposite direction. You may find painful muscle that is stretched and pulling the vertebra causing muscular pains in the involved areas, range of motion limitation, headaches, and numbness or tingling in the arms or hands.

A good way to determine which short-leg syndrome you may have. There is a test known as the Deerfield Test. With the person lying face down, check the length by correcting any pronation or supination of the feet so that the heels are parallel and perpendicular to the plane of the legs. This may be easier to tell with shoes on. The heel has a straight edge and may be obvious to compare it with the plane of the table rather than bare feet.

After determining which leg is short, flex both knees to 90°. If it is anatomical shortness, the difference in leg length will not change in positions 1 and 2, that is extended or bent to 90 degrees. If it is a functional shortness, the short leg will appear to become longer as the other or normal leg or longer when in the flex position. If it is functional shortness, the short leg will be either become as long as the other leg or longer when in the flex position. Whichever syndrome one is suffering from, the weight will be uneven as it is distributed between both legs.

There are some red flags that may show up to help determine if this patient is anatomical of functional short leg syndrome. If the pain is exaggerated by running, associated with low back pain, perhaps ankle and foot pain, and if the same muscle is pulled or injured repeatedly, shin splints, sciatic pain, hip muscle discomfort, are all common problems.

How does a functional leg-length difference develop? Over a number of years you find yourself doing repetitive motion at your job from leaning on the same side with rotation or turning, always carrying things with the same arm and leaning to compensate, carrying children, or if you sleep on the same side every night, or even the delivery when you were born from forceps may be a factor.

Sometimes you can see the difference in your side in a photograph, leaning to one side or a shoulder higher than the other or maybe the head is tilted to balance out the frame. You may even find that the hem in you slacks ride higher than the other leg. Sometimes runners notice that the longer leg feels more impact when they run and sends a shock up the spine. The longer leg will see the heel of the shoe wear prematurely.

When you determine if the shorter leg is a result of anatomical all you need to do is insert a heel lift to make up the difference between both legs. The difference can be compensated by inserting "Dr. Scholls" foot pads into the shoe of the short side.

Functional shortness is more complicated. The has to be a reason for this condition. A functional leg-length discrepancy is present in 60 percent of people. The difference can be small or very great. If there is a minimal difference, there are usually no obvious pain, from it. In time, however, a minimal difference always becomes compounds itself and becomes greater. Since the impact in a runner is more, the change is much more rapid. In the runner, there is usually a more rapid change in leg length, as running involves tremendous vertical impact. Gravity eventually wins if nothing is done to correct the imbalance.

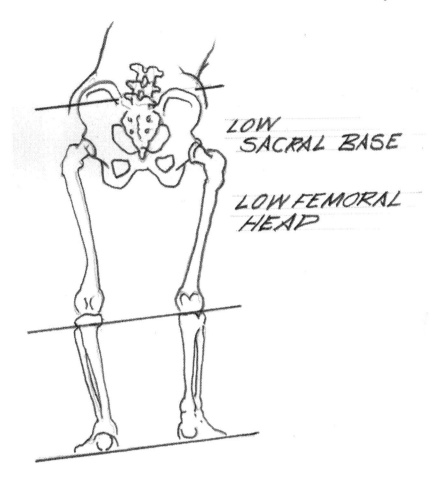

Maybe some of the reasons are: (1) One of the arches is different. (correction can be done with the arch supports or orthotics). (2) Perhaps one of the joints in the knee, hip or ankle has a different range of motion. All of the joints involved should be checked to make sure they are synchronized with both sides including ankle, knee, hip, and low back, should be put through a full range of motion to ensure normal equal motion. (3) A weakness in one of the lower extremity muscles which can pull the torso forward, an imbalance of each side prohibiting synchronization of the pelvis to rotate either anterior (forward) or posterior (backward) in relationship to the other side. (4) Bad habits, such as bad posture, slouching in chairs, carrying a heavy load like a tool box on the same side for long periods of time, crossing legs while sitting, standing with all your weight on one leg, always running on the same side of a beveled roads or insufficient stretching.

(5) Poor quality running shoes.

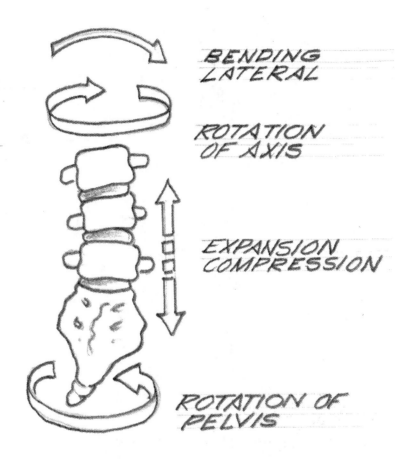

BENDING LATERAL

ROTATION OF AXIS

EXPANSION COMPRESSION

ROTATION OF PELVIS

To fix or repair functional shortness involves a number of factors. First, correction of any structural faults has to be changed or removed to allow for even out the weight distribution and normal movement of the joint and muscle involved. Change any hypertrophied or tight muscles that cause imbalances (right vs. left and front vs. back) that become apparent after a through kinesiological examination by a qualified chiropractor. After changing the muscles that are not evenly toned, manipulation of the involved joints by a chiropractor is performed to correct any structural subluxations. This restores all the joints to function under a normal weight balance. Second, observe the patient walk at a slow gate and perhaps run. Sometimes the leans to compensate for these discrepancies such as one arm held close to the body in its correct motion

The frequency of injury is much less when the body is lined up and the joints will last longer. On the first visit find out the amount of difference between the legs, try to restore normal alignment. It will take about 4 weeks for the change to reach half way to the correction and be evident. The younger the patient is the quicker you will see results. Develop some stretches for the patient to help the muscles develop new muscle memories and maintain their new assignments.

CHAPTER 22

Frozen SI Joint

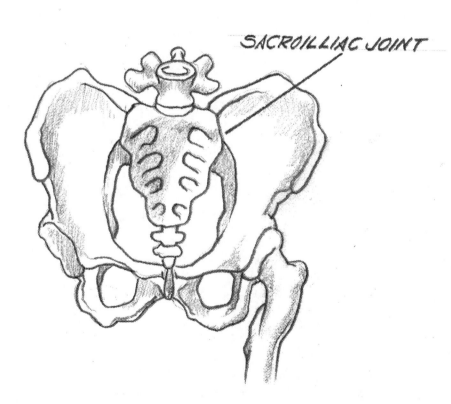

SACROILLIAC JOINT

Checking for a frozen SI joint can be done by having your patient stand with their back to you, place their feet a foot apart, and bend forward letting the arms hang. The therapist places each thumb on the dimples of the lumbar or the articulation point of the two bones, (sacrum an iliac) where they meet. If either thumb rises up when they bend that is the location where the frozen joint is. The sacrum and the iliac should move independently in relationship to each other. If your thumb rises up on either side that joint is frozen.

Pain located either to the left or right of your lower ack.

The pain can range from an ache to a sharp pain which can restrict movement.

- The pain may move out into your Gluteal muscles in the hip and back and will often radiate to the front into the groin. In some cases it may be the reason for pain in the testicles in males.
- Sometimes there is discomfort that could even be misdiagnosed as sciatica because of the evidence of pain going down the legs.
- If you have a problem getting in or out of the car, putting on your socks and shoes or turning in bed, these could be symptoms of a frozen SI joint. If you experience tightness after long rides in the car or getting out of bed this joint should be looked at.

Frozen Shoulder Syndrome;

When your patient cant comb their hair or experiences difficulty using the arms to dress you will find problems in the deltoid, brachial and some of the tissues on the opposite side in the upper back area. I have not seen this condition occur in both shoulder at the same time. I have seen this problem more often in patients over 40 and even more in females. After finding the trigger point or hot spot bend the arm at the elbow and raise the elbow up so the hand of the patient is resting on the trapezoid. The patient may be surprised that they can raise their arm that far. Explain that your muscle moved it and not theirs so it did not contract to cause the pain but rather you put the arm in this position so that the fibers of the deltoid are in their resting state and will release easier. As you raise the elbow up slowly make small rotational circles with the elbow which sends another signal to the brain. The more slight movements you execute the less chance it will hurt because the brain can only read one signal coming from that location and will not perceive the pain. Use deep tissue pressure with a slight slide to it. Finish up with sliding friction up towards the heart.

If your patient has made an appointment chances are you will be asked to remove their pain. You could be forced to deal with conditions that you can only contribute to the end result and may need to work in conjunction with a doctor as a team. Certain types of pain may require surgery and you need to inform the patient that what you have to offer is a temporary reduction of the pain by removing the edema. Debilitating pain may require treatment plans as a team. Yet in the case of severe pain, how true is the old adage about prevention being better than a cure? For many patients suffering from pain, there is no relief in these sentiments. For many modern conditions, the cause hasn't been precisely pinned down, making prevention a difficult science. Just like fibromyalgia, frozen shoulder syndrome isn't well understood by the medical community.

Evaluate your patient by checking both sides of the body, make note of the muscle tissues involved, and check range of motion and pain levels during movement. Work as deep as you can without ca\using too much pain. One method you can try is movement within the existing travel of the limb until you reach restriction. Try raising the arm while making small circles, and then add a bouncing movement while all the time increasing the range. The brain can only carry one message at a time to the brain and that is ouch. When you confuse the brain by sending several other messages like the different movements you are creating there is no room for ouch and you sometimes see more direction in the range.

CHAPTER 23

Muscle Testing:

Kinesiology is another word for muscle testing. Muscle testing is a simple test to tell what your body's needs are. Since we all have electrical systems all of us can do it. When observing this method it just looks too simple and many assume it is a parlor trick or gimmick. Your body needs electric to make the synapse spark to move muscle, make your heart beat and much more. This electrical field can be photographed with infra-red film.

Your chiropractor or holistic physician are experienced and schooled in muscle testing. You have pathways of electrical current surging throughout your body. These pathways are called meridians. Every body part has its own separate meridian and it needs to stay in balance. When this current is disrupted weakness in the body part is the result. When the doctor asks you to extend your arm, and resist the downward motion when he tries to push it down he is muscle testing you. Your other hand is holding a supplement to your chest. If this supplement is what your body needs, your arm will be strong and he cant push it down. If the item is not good for your condition it will weaken the arm and drop readily downward.

You can test yourself if you need to know if your body needs a mineral, vitamin, or product to enhance a problem that you have noticed try to put your thumb and little finger of the same hand together. If you are right handed do this with the left hand. and vice versa if you are left handed. This creates a closed circuit from your body. It has the ability to answer yes or no when you hold the product in question next to your chest. If the product in question is a good thing it will cause the closed circuit to create a negative energy and weaken the fingers allowing someone to pull them apart very easily. If. its a good thing for your body, it will create positive energy and you will find your fingers very strong and difficult for your helper to pull apart. Keep in mind that the circuit you created with your fingers is a temporary circuit for the purpose of testing and not being used for any body function or activity. Yet the current status of your body's imbalance is and extension of the rest of the body. The yes or no answer you receive is over and beyond what you perceive or think in your brain, it is your body telling you what it needs.

Infant Massage:

What are the benefits of infant massage?

- Relaxes Infant
  Babies experience stress and it is obvious when they get fussy and irritable. Properly done it releases gas and aids in colic. A gentle loving touch is a basic human need and is desired at the beginning of life.
- Improves Bonding
  A gentle touch identifies the parent with a nurturing and love connection, its the basic building block for forming emotional and healthy body growth.
- Helps body Growth and Development
  Tests have shown weight gain is improved and immune function. Nerve development is enhanced which extends to the brain and muscle growth.
- Establishes Communication
  Mom and Dad learn and observe visual and verbal sounds the baby makes.
- Baby's Sleep is improved
  Your baby will look forward to this time. As the massage removes stress the pathway for a restful sleep is established and perhaps longer periods of sleep.

We have been studying the benefits of infant massage since the 1970's and evidence says babies born premature, drug babies and babies with complications all benefit from massage. Their appetite is improved; sleep patterns, less digestive problems, and even better weight gain.

Some therapists specialize with this new approach to massage and build a good practice up with this specialty. Some of the more progressive hospitals use infant massage to help the newborn finish the birthing process if they entered the world by caesarian method. Without the contractions of the birth canal neural pathways are not established correctly and have shown to be a problem later on in life.

There are a lot of the common ailments and diseases that you may encounter with your patients. I have listed some of them and there are volumes of books that address them. I felt a brief description of what they are would help and suggested treatment procedures and the role that massage therapy can do for them

Asthma

Aromatherapy massage

Is helpful when using essential oils like eucalyptus, lemon, Himalayan cedar wood, and others to rub into the face, neck, and chest areas. These oils will unlock nasal passages, and loosen phlegm to improve breathing. Sometimes percussion strokes by cupping your hands and repeatedly pounding around the rib cage and Mediasteinum area will help to expel congestion fluids. Massage should be done in the intercostals and from the top of the chest in a downwards direction.

CHAPTER 24

Disorders and diseases that massage may help

Reynaud's Syndrome

Reynaud's is a rare disorder that affects the arteries. Reynaud's is sometimes called a disease, a syndrome, or phenomenon. The disorder is noted by short periods of vasospasm (narrowing of the blood vessels).

You can help combat vasospasm of the arteries or reduces blood flow to the fingers and toes. In people who have Reynaud's, by massaging the calves and feet and hands and forearm.

Cohn's Disease

How does massage therapy benefit Cohn's sufferers? Cohn's disease creates a lot of stress and will often make the condition worse. Many tests have shown that massage reduces the stress Studies, conducted on massage therapy as treatment for Cohn's disease symptoms. Massage can reduce the symptoms and pain associated with this disease.

Gout:

A lot of people do not realize that gout is a form of arthritis. Gout is caused by a build-up of a waste product, uric acid, in the bloodstream. Uric acid is one of the body's waste products. Normally it is dissolved in the bloodstream, filtered out by the kidneys and excreted in urine. However a build-up of uric acid may settle in the joints in the form of crystals, causing inflammation and pain. This is called gout.

The joint of the big toe is usually the first site to experience an attack. The toe becomes red, swollen and extremely painful. Other joints commonly affected include the knee, ankle and those of the feet. Gout strikes most people at the age of 40 to 50 and are predominately males. During full blown gout attach or shortly after one it is too painful to do massage on your patient. Gently massage the foot using lots of joint movement in the ankle and toes. To break up the crystals formed in the joint and follow with friction. A good natural addition to your treatment is to suggest black cherry juice to help neutralize the uric acid and reduce the pain.

Bells Palsy:

Sometimes a person can wake up with this sudden onset disorder. There will usually experience discomfort and pain behind the ear and extending down to the sub-occipital. There is a numbness to the face and the patient will note an eyelid and or mouth with less control and a marked visual change than the unaffected opposite side. The face droops on the affected side and sometimes slurred speech with less expression.

Make sure that your patient did not have a stroke before moving forward on treatment. We are unsure of the cause for Bells Palsy. We feel that it is association with Cranial Nerve VII. There may an inflammation or infection causing this condition that is affecting the nerve. I have seen most patients recover from Bells Palsy within a few weeks.

In the face, the skin is attached to the muscles hence we get our fascial expressions. Work on the affected side of the face and do basic face massage techniques by rolling the skin, lifting stretching the muscles and rotating it. I also try to release the Pterygoid lateral inside the mouth. Work along the temple near the ear where the blood flow enters, do the cheeks, and along the temple. At the end of the session, there is an area at the base of the skull under the sub-occipital ridge outer edge. This is a very convenient Acupressure point that sometimes helps. Bells Palsy. Massage will increase the blood flow to nourish the nerves and muscles involved.

What is Thoracic Outlet Syndrome?

Though many people with this condition cant remember what they did to cause this problem other than think they may have just "slept wrong" and awakened with a numb hand. Thoracic Outlet Syndrome is the name given to a group of painful nerve impingements. Sometimes heavy lifting injury, sitting for long periods at a desk, or sports may cause the muscles in the neck (scalene, trapezium, and infra spinatis. Patients complain of discomfort and pain in the wrist and arm. Try to remember there is usually a restriction of blood flow that needs to be addressed also.

There are a number of causes for Thoracic Outlet Syndrome including whiplash injuries from motor vehicle accidents and sports injuries. Postural issues, especially a forward head posture like that maintained by office workers and computer users, can also trigger the onset of this syndrome. Thoracic Outlet Syndrome may also be the result of overstressing the muscles in the thoracic outlet area during exercise, or by impact injuries to the shoulder or upper chest area. Additionally, though it is rare, a "cervical rib" may be the blame for this condition.

Massage Therapy and Bodywork for Thoracic Outlet Syndrome

You can approach treatment using Neuromuscular Therapy, Trigger Point Therapy, and Deep Tissue Myotherapy. I feel that all of these methods overlap each other and are similar. I approach with the deep tissue method. I check range of motion of the affected side and search for trigger points to release and stretch. I systematically one by one search all the muscle tissue in the deltoid, neck front and back then the upper back. Check the Pectoralis minor, Brachii and scalene in the area. Your goal is to release and lengthen fibers and remove the pressure from the nerves.

Sometimes this condition will keep the patient from sleeping throughout the night. Instruct the patient to raise his arm on the affected side and put his hand behind his head then let the elbow drop. This removes the pressure from the nerves by repositioning or relaxing the muscle causing the numbness.

Shin splints

This reason for this condition often involves tearing or traumatized soft tissues on the front of the shin. There are two groups of muscles along the tibia. The location of the pain depends on which group of muscles is damaged.

The pain experienced usually is on the front outside edge of the shin. Another place is the middle of the tibia. This pain is sharp and is usually goes along the tibia when you run or perform some type of aggressive sport that flexes the ankle greatly with a lot change of direction, quick stopping or jumping. It can be caused by training on blacktop or concrete pushing your training too far, or too much running uphill and downhill. If you have an injury in the abs or gluteus core muscles the shins may pay for the overworked body movement.

The muscles and their tendons become swollen and the bones themselves where they grow out of cause the bones to hurt also. The anterior tibia and fibula become tender to the touch and actually hurt all the time until repaired.

Anterolateral shin splints

This means the front and outside of the Tibia hurts. All of your body weight is transferred to the heel in each step to stop the downward movement of the body and push with the balls of the same foot. You will also notice an increase in pain if you keep using it or increase the distance.

Posteromedial shin splints

This type of shin splint will show up in the low back side of the leg, and seems to be deeper.

The Tibialis supports the arch of the foot as when the body moves over the foot as you step to the ground. If the arch is not supported by a good pair of shoes, Posteromedial shin splints is most likely the result. If this is not attended to the foot could turn into a flat foot condition, resulting from the Hyperpronation.

Treatment options:

Stop running! These muscles need to have time to heal. Do a non load bearing activity, like swimming or ride a bike. Begin your treatment by reducing the swelling. I use moist heat to dilate the capillaries of the traumatized muscle for 3 min. and then apply ice for 30 seconds. This process dilates the vessels to 300 % to allow blood flow to enter, remove wastes, brings in repair material, anti-histamine, brings into the area endorphins to help with the pain. Repeat the hot and cold about 10 times starting and ending with the moist heat. This method speeds up the healing 3 times faster. It is important to use moist heat instead of a dry heat Dry heat pulls the blood away from the affected area to the surface. This opening and closing of the tissue creates a pumping action like a massage on the cellular level. The metabolic action speeds up the healing.

After using the hot and cold revolutions, its time for massage and can be done every other day. Remember you are dealing with overused muscles to loosen up and stretch. There is nothing like massage to reverse this condition. For both types of shin splints, concentrate on loosening the tendons and remove edema. Do light stretching and bring in lots of blood. Make sure you attend to all of the muscles in the lower leg front and back.

Drop Foot

If you can't walk on your heels without difficulty it's a good indication you have this condition. Weakening of the ankle flexors or in the toes is the reason for this condition, causing the person to drag the front of the foot. You will note that the person needs to raise his knee higher because the front of the foot drops down if not high enough and drags.

Drop foot is the result of damage to the nerve originating in the lower back. This neuromuscular disorder can sometimes be alleviated by deep tissue release of the impinging soft tissues causing the condition. Sometimes deep tissue can release the impingement at the origin of the nerve in the spine. Improvement sometimes is noted if the pressure is released on the peroneal nerve. If there is a bulging disc involved light massage may release the swelling of the nucleus pulpous enough for it to recede back. Other conditions that are more serious and requires surgery should be dealt with by a surgeon.

Scoliosis

The spine has curves in it, the primary and secondary curves that develop when we are infants and raise our torso and neck up to develop them. When there is a abnormal curve one of these conditions is diagnosed as scoliosis.

Deep Tissue Massage—Deep tissue work, and assisted stretching techniques to hypertrophic muscles, improve local circulation; can reduce muscular pain and related fascia. When you relax the tight muscles pulling the spine too far and balance the soft tissues on each side of the spinal column there can be noted correction. The steady pulling of the muscles constantly pulls the vertebra and may cause breathing problems and sleeping issues. I have never considered scoliosis to be a bone problem but a soft tissue issue.

Relaxation of the tight muscles involved will allow the spine to balance out itself along the vertical axis. There is no such thing as a perfect spine. Everyone has some sort of scoliosis, Lordosis, or Kipsies to some degree. If you look at the slight deviations of the spinal column it could be a key for diagnosing some of the muscle pain in the back.

Bone spurs

Bone spurs are usually caused by extreme pressure of the attachment of the muscles tendon. The brain compensates by building up or re-enforcement of the bone with calcium deposits to strengthen the attachment. The Calcanial bone or heal bone is the only place on the body that massage therapy can alleviate a spur condition. This is caused by the Achilles tendon attachment is strained by the Gastronomies Muscle being too tight. If surgery is done the spur usually returns because the reason for its existence is not removed. Stretching this muscle and the other calf muscles will remove the tension on the bone and remedy this condition.

Degenerative Disc Disease

As we get older we get shorter because of the disc weakening and becoming thinner. As the spacing between the vertebra becomes less the nerves that exit between them from the spinal column become compressed. Nerve compression is the result of walking upright with constant pounding of the body's weight every step we take over the years causing pain and tightness of the back.

When you do massage therapy, the pressure applied, evenly distributes the pain by interrupting the Krebs pain cycle of muscles tightening. Blood circulation to the soft tissues and the disc improves the integrity of the involved tissues thus slowing down the development of the condition. You may experience some relief for your patient with the use of trigger point therapy on the hot spots and release of the tight muscles which improves range of motion as well.

Parkinson's disease:

Your patient suffers from tremors especially in the hand when it is not holding anything. You will not that they write very tiny and lean forward and shuffle when they walk. Muscles become ridged and posture changes are noted. Production of a chemical called dopamine from the brain that helps muscle movement is reduced or limited. Dopamine is produced in other parts of the body but is restricted to the area needed in the brain because the blood brain barrier prevents entry. This disease is progressive but drug treatment slows down the progression.

Because the muscles are tight in a Parkinson's patient it is up to you to relax the tightness, help improve the range of motion, bring into the limbs new blood. Massage will help remove the toxins and help with the tired exhausted from the constant battle of dealing with this disease. When you massage these tissues it brings into the area endorphins to relax and help with the pain. The blood is increased 3 times with Swedish work. Try stretching the muscles to make the tendons and ligaments longer Joint movements are helpful to try to preserve the range of motion integrity as long as possible.

Massage will help with the spasms and generally make the patient feel better.

Muscular Dystrophy

This muscle condition causes the muscle tissues to tighten and pull on the joints to the point where movement is limited. Deformity develops and mobility becomes very limited along with circulation that is lessoned. Patients develop mental problems along with their pain. Swedish and deep tissue work will help this problem. Work on the range of motion to slow down deformity. Concentrate on lengthening the muscle involved.

Fibromyalgia:

Probably one of the most misdiagnosed conditions today. Fibromyalgia is an easy diagnosis for unexplained pain and discomfort for doctors to use today and has become a great "buzz word". If the patient has the 11 hot spots of discomfort in the neck, shoulder, and chest areas it seems it is a sure thing. However, there are no tests available to verify the disease. Fibromyalgia will not release when you apply acupressure to these painful sites. If it releases then it is only tight traumatized muscle fiber that needed attention.

Fibromyalgia makes you to hurt all over. You will feel fatigued and like you never have enough sleep. Body parts will hurt to the touch and swollen. Parts of your body will hurt to move and to touch them. Your muscles may feel like they have been overworked or pulled. Excessive exercise is out of the question, and the simplest task seems overwhelming. The patient will experience depression, headaches, dry mouth, sensitivity to heat or cold, fogginess of the brain, tingling and partial numbness in the appendages.

There are no specific laboratory tests to diagnose fibromyalgia. Sometimes the body manufactures fibroblast cells. These fibroblast cells make up the structure of ligaments, tendons, and bone. These cells look like slivers of glass and are very rigid. This is where the strength of the bones comes from. These cells are created in pockets and develop in soft tissue for some unexplained reason. As the fibers of the muscle slide through them it is very uncomfortable causing the pain we feel in fibromyalgia. These cells are bone cell in character it is listed in the arthritis diseases and is number three of over 200 types of arthritis.

I have treated many patients diagnosed with fibromyalgia and after locating the site of pain, it will release after deep tissue work is applied. Fibromyalgia will not release but needs to be broken up. This tells me it was initially only traumatized muscle tissue that needed to be released and not fibromyalgia.

Frozen Shoulder Syndrome:

In acute situations, the use of ice packs will be useful. Determine the range of motion as a reference point. Examine the Deltoid for hot spots, the Pictorial muscles, and Scapula. Use friction to bring blood into the areas that you find and gradually deep kneading. Gently raise the arm testing your progress and add additional movements like slow circular motion while pumping slightly up and down. These multiple movements are multiple impulses to the brain. The nerves of the Brachial Plexus can only carry one signal at a time and the patient sometimes does not feel the discomfort as you pass the reference point of range of motion previously noted.

Bronchitis:

You want to reduce the symptoms by dislodging the mucus from the bronchi. Vigorous chest cupping on the rib cage on the front, sides and back will help loosen the mucus. Advise your female patients to use their hands to cover the breast area and move them to the side to be more effective with your cupping percussion technique. Clients suffering with this problem are prone to repertory infection and if the patient has a mild form of infection reschedule as to not infect others.

Carpal Tunnel Syndrome:

This condition is sometimes misdiagnosed and relief can be gained if the Brachial Plexus is not impinged. Check all the muscles around the Scapula and upper back. The Deltoid muscles and neck muscles should all be released to verify there is no Brachial Plexus impingement.

Constipation:

Position the patient in the supine position and instruct them to bend their knees. Place a pillow under the hips. Proceed to do deep tissue kneading of the abdominal area pushing and rolling the viscera back and forth. After loading the area with new blood and relaxing the general area you proceed to massage the colon. The colon massage is started on the base of the ascending colon. Use your right hand fingers to push down at this point. Use the left hand to push down beside the other and slowly make small circular movements while moving up the colon to the junction of the beginning of the transverse colon. Do not lift your left hand. Remember that you are moving the contents of the colon and do not want the contents to slide back. You move the right hand up beside the left hand and proceed to go across the transverse colon while making small circular movements until you reach the beginning of the descending colon. Do not raise your hand and continue the pressure. Continue with the left hand down the descending colon in the same manner. The procedure is referred to as the Zablowdowski Technique, and if done several times it will empty a stubborn colon. This method should not be used on patients suffering from diverticulitis, cancer in the general area, or recent surgery of the abdominal area.

CHAPTER 25

Hair Analysis:

This process is a great diagnostic tool for any massage business. You can analyze your patient's mineral content for deficiency. The enzymes in your body cannot function without minerals. If your patient suffers from some difficulty with no obvious reason you can check mineral loss and correct the deficiency. Signs of mineral deficiency are white spots on the nails to indicate zinc loss, ridges indicate an iron loss, if you have an calcium and or copper loss your nails and hair will be brittle. If you notice deep groves across the nail this means your patient needs calcium. Stretch marks show a loss of calcium. Zink deficiency will cause growth loss in younger people. When the body builds up toxic metal such as lead, mercury, or cadmium there will be mood swings and dramatic emotional changes. These can accumulate from the job site as well. Hair sample analysis can be an individual screening for you patient's individual needs. Mineral imbalances can cause depression, hypoglycemia, headaches, and stress.

You can secure the services of a lab specializing in this service. Send in hair sample and a small fee is paid. Within a few days the results can be faxed to your office with all of the results. Hair analysis can determine exactly what vitamins you need. Did you know that BP and strokes may be the result of too much sodium chloride; migraines may be the result of too much copper and iron, proper zinc level regulate sugar, multiple sclerosis is linked to high iron content, and magnesium deficiency is linked to epilepsy, leukemia, heart disease, and kidney problems. Manic depression is caused by high levels of lithium. Hair analysis is as useful as an executive profile blood test.

Marketing your skills:

Therapeutic medical massage contributes a lot to today's alternative health care. In addition to the pain relief you offer in your office, why not add some other choices such as massage for relaxation, facial massage, foot massage, ear candling, exfoliation massage, body wraps, or a paraffin dip to soothe the feet or hands. Consider adding a steam sauna, Jacuzzi or a tanning booth. Combo packs to use as a gift certificate for that someone special. Couples massage is a good way to introduce massage to someone who is reluctant to get a massage but will try it when someone joins them as a couple, for example, a friend, a family member, or a spouse beside them. In this case you would need an extra table and another therapist to assist you.

CHAPTER 26

Herbs:

Every therapist should have knowledge of the basic healing qualities of the herbs that grow on this mother earth. There are some basic truths that seem to follow through with these plants. If you look at the root of most tonics, they are shaped like the human body, since the tonics treats the entire body. Most plants with a yellow flower are good for the urinary track, plants with a red blossom are good for the blood stream and heart, plants with a white flower are usually great for disinfection, plants that grow with a thorn usually help pain, and plants that grow in cold damp areas are good for colds.

Plants are grouped into different classes depending on how they help the body. These categories would include: Stimulants, Diuretics, Expectorants, Astringents, Nervines, and Tonics

Stimulants: These herbs excite the systems of the body and promote increased blood circulation. Examples would be most mints, cloves, anise, sage, red clover, ginger root, rosemary, comfrey, ginseng, cayenne pepper, and lemon balm, to name a few.

Diuretics: These plants help to detoxify the body by increasing urine flow. Examples would be parsley, burdock, nettle, dandelion, apples, anise, corn silk, and red raspberry.

Expectorants: These herbs help to break up mucus remove it from the chest. Examples of a expectorant would be slippery elm, ginger, garlic, horse radish, anise, lemon balm, lobelia, and wild cherry bark.

Astringents: Herbs that are in this class cleanse the body and also act as antibiotic. Some good examples of astringents would be witch hazel, thyme, mints of all types, nettle, sweet basil, sage, rosemary, eyebright, willow bark, and lemon balm.

Nervines: These herbs relax the nervous system like the following plants, hops, chamomile, basil, red clover, willow, valerian, yarrow, rosemary, and catnip.

Tonics: Enhances and strengthens all the systems supported by the digestion system. A good tonic would be dandelion, rosemary, parsley, goldenseal, sassafras, ginger, ginsing, anise, nettle, hops, and white yarrow.

Networking is promoting you. Use the newspapers and radio for advertisement, run specials for the purpose of increased cliental, consider an open house to educate the public. Network! Get out there and mingle take part in community activities. Let the public get to know you by getting involved.

Malpractice Insurance

Something to consider: Be aware of your legal scope of practice. What are your limitations as to diagnostic procedure, legally what can you advise, and remember that you are not a doctor without the training and certifications.

Code of Ethics,

Establish a good code of ethics to follow. Fair business practices. Charge a fair price for a quality service.

Should you fly solo or hook up with a doctor or chiropractor? Perhaps work in a spa or hair design business? If you are by yourself, you will have much more free reign but more overhead. If you are connected with a doctor, you will need to work under the jurisdiction of the physician and your practice may be limited.

Some of the benefits are insurance may pay for your patients treatments if your doctor is writing scripts for your services. The combination of massage and spinal adjustment from the chiropractor is a very aggressive form of treatment. You also need to ask yourself if the doctor you are associated with believe in what you do or is it just to gain on the competition and add to his marketing. One angle to look at is that most likely you will have the loyalty of the doctor's patients but not be referred to by the other doctors in town. Being an independent therapist allows you to be available to the general public without infringing on clientele of just one office. Will your patients take you more serious if you are associated with a beauty salon? Does your practice tailor itself towards beauty and spa treatment or is it geared towards the medical field? You may consider taking on a partner and share the work load. Sometimes another person allows you more flexibility for sick time or vacation while keeping your office open. Someone extra to answer the phone when you are with a patient, share the overhead expenses, and flexible hours. You may find that you each have your strong points and are able to offer more variety to the public.

Different therapists have different styles. Some have a heavier hand, some like to do relaxation techniques as opposed to medical therapeutic techniques. Different strokes for different folks!

You should consider attending continuing education in the areas that you may be interested in around your area. The more tools that you have in your tool box the more resources you have at hand to accomplish successful treatments.

If you want to appear more professional you should consider a laundry service for your towels, sheets and pillow cases. Another nice addition would be a receptionist.

CHAPTER 27

Muscle charts

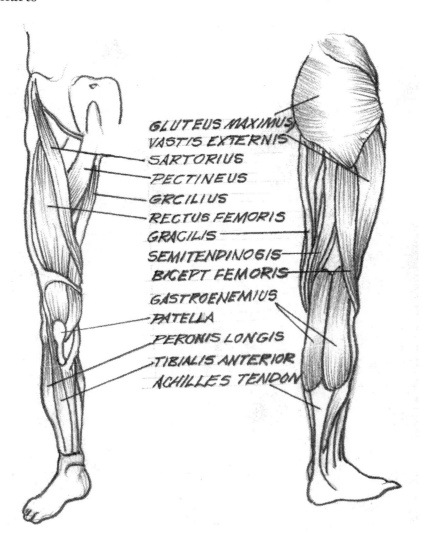

GLUTEUS MAXIMUS
VASTIS EXTERNIS
SARTORIUS
PECTINEUS
GRCILIUS
RECTUS FEMORIS
GRACILIS
SEMITENDINOGIS
BICEPT FEMORIS
GASTROENEMIUS
PATELLA
PERONIS LONGIS
TIBIALIS ANTERIOR
ACHILLES TENDON

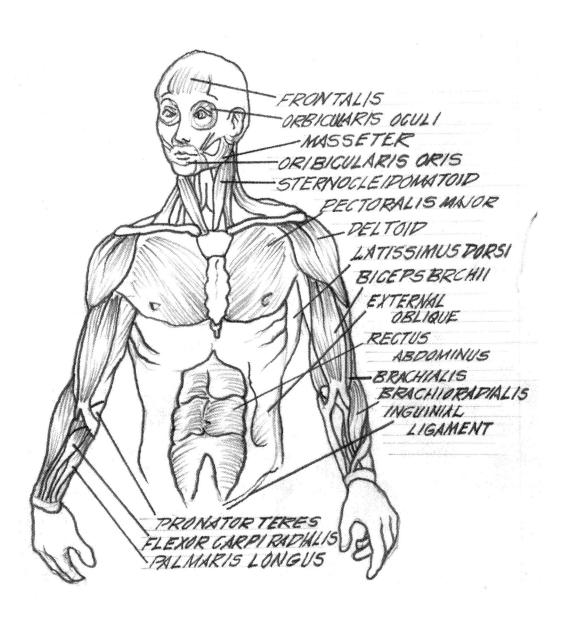

FRONTALIS
ORBICUARIS OCULI
MASSETER
ORIBICULARIS ORIS
STERNOCLEIDOMATOID
PECTORALIS MAJOR
DELTOID
LATISSIMUS DORSI
BICEPS BRCHII
EXTERNAL
    OBLIQUE
RECTUS
    ABDOMINUS
BRACHIALIS
BRACHIORADIALIS
INGUINIAL
    LIGAMENT

PRONATOR TERES
FLEXOR CARPI RADIALIS
PALMARIS LONGUS

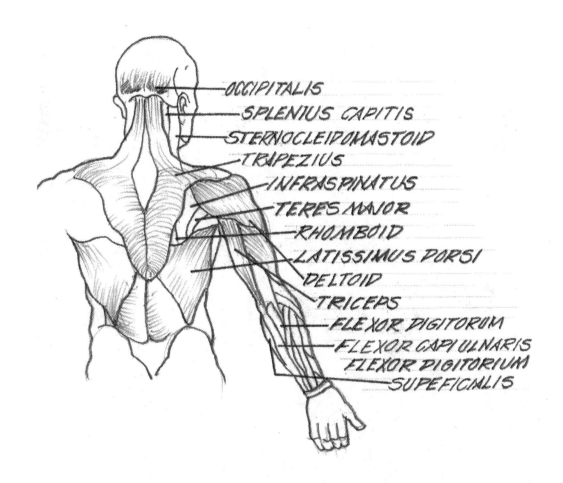

OCCIPITALIS

SPLENIUS CAPITIS

STERNOCLEIDOMASTOID

TRAPEZIUS

INFRASPINATUS

TERES MAJOR

RHOMBOID

LATISSIMUS DORSI

DELTOID

TRICEPS

FLEXOR DIGITORUM

FLEXOR CAPI ULNARIS

FLEXOR DIGITORIUM

SUPEFICALIS